ProMetabolics

YOUR PERSONAL GUIDE to TRANSFORMATIONAL HEALTH and HEALING

Humbart "Smokey" Santillo, N.D.

DESIGNS FOR WELLNESS PRESS
CARLSBAD, CALIFORNIA © 2008

Cover Illustration by Oliver Burston   Cover Design by George Foster
www.DebutArt.com   www.FosterCovers.com

Index by Madge Walls, *All Sky Indexing*

Other publications by Dr. Santillo:
Herbal Combinations from Authoritative Sources
Natural Healing with Herbs
Natural Healing Herbal Correspondence Course
Intuitive Eating: Everybody's Guide to Lifelong Health and Vitality Through Food
The Basics of Intuitive Eating
Food Enzymes: The Missing Link to Radiant Health

Visit Dr. Santillo's Web site at: www.SmokeySantillo.com

Pro · Met · a · bol · ics
[**Pro**-Met-*uh*-**bol**-iks]

Promoting processes which enhance
and optimize metabolic functions
of the human body

Edited by Kate B. Johnson, B.A.
and Roy E. Vartabedian, Dr.P.H.

DEDICATION

This book is dedicated to all of the Juice Plus+® distributors around the world. My two children, Jessica Marie and Nicholas James, and I would like to personally thank each and every one of you for making so many wonderful things possible in our lives.

Stay well.

– Dr. Humbart "Smokey" Santillo

pH paper:
Micro Essential Lab - 718-338-3618
Berts Pharmacy - 570-888-2157

Mountain States Health Products
plant derived - all 4 types
amylase, protease, lipase, cellulase

ACKNOWLEDGEMENTS

I'm so fortunate to have these people in my life.

Dr. Roy Vartabedian, my publisher. I'd like to thank him for doing such a great job. He worked so quickly and efficiently and put together a great team. The best to his wife, Renée, and their son, my new friend Alex.

Kio Atkinson, thanks for so much love and support. And a special "Hi" to her genius daughter, Darbie Atkinson.

Thanks to Kate Johnson, my editor, who did a wonderful job with the manuscript. I enjoyed working with you and look forward to working together on future books.

Thanks to Oliver Burston and George Foster, who did a brilliant job of designing and illustrating the concept of *ProMetabolics* on our cover.

Thanks to Madge Walls, who did a very professional job of putting together the index of the book.

Thanks to NSA corporate—Jay Martin, John Blair, and Charlie Evans—for their support. Thanks to Elton Dubose, your support has always been special to me. I would also like to give a special thanks to NSA's Randy Mathews and Yvette Sanders for thinking out of the box.

Diane and Dr. Frank Torelli, D.C., are great friends, and Frank is a pristine chiropractor in Alden, New York.

Tony Collier, owner of the National Enzyme Company. I'll never forget how Tony spent five hours a day for two years on the phone with me while I had some health challenges. You got me through, Tony.

Mike Barnhart, my friend and working partner with Juice Plus+®.

Frank and Dawn Berrafato. Frank and I have been training together for more than twenty years. I love both of you.

Cindy Grogan, for typing out the manuscript.

Dr. Richard Gerow.

Dan McCue and his lady, Sharon. Dan has always been there.

Charles Spillman.

Brother Mike Santillo and family: Anna, Elaina, and Mary.

Dr. Mitra Ray, Ph.D. Thanks for mentioning my name from the stage.

Timothy Speciale, D.O., a great friend and prolotherapist in Williamsville, New York, a true healer (866-692-2723).

Sharon Lynn, owner of Mountain States Health Products, Inc. Your knowledge, friendship, and wisdom in healing are special.

Ryan Falzone. We love and miss you.

The Tinder Boys.

Scott and Jody Kupinger, neighbors and Skipper's best friends.

Scott McCarthy, pristine accountant and friend.

Dr. Debbie Patrick, mentor and naturopath in Tucson, Arizona. We think alike.

Dr. Morris Zubkewych, D.C., a tremendous healer and great friend. I can't think of when I couldn't count on you. Live forever, Morris, the world needs you.

Dave and Patricia Malin.

Paul Childress and Ryan Groneman, my personal trainers extraordinaire. Paul and Ryan are the top trainers at the University of Buffalo's Sports Performance Center and well-known power lifters.

Dr. Riyaz Hassanali, M.D. Great friend and tops in dermatologic cosmetic surgery in Williamsville, New York.

Jeff Roberti. Thank you, Jeff, for having intuitive sense when I first told you about Juice Plus+®. Jeff set me up for the first meeting with NSA.

TABLE OF CONTENTS

FOREWORD

First, let me start off by saying it is a genuine honor to have the opportunity to contribute to Dr. Smokey Santillo's new book. I have known Smokey for more than fifteen years and consider him a friend as well as a business associate. I know him as a pioneer in his field, a talented businessman, a great athlete, and a loving father. I have seen him touch and change the lives of millions of people through his products and his educational endeavors.

Smokey and I have worked together on various projects over the years. He is one of the unique individuals you meet in life who has a higher level of understanding about his area of expertise. Smokey has a gift for generating new ideas, products, strategies, and solutions in the area of alternative medicine. His insights and contributions are changing the face of healthcare today. Smokey has always been that unique professional who can not only study and apply the insights of others, but more importantly, can create and apply so many new ones of his own.

My history with Smokey began when he met an associate of my business partner, Jeff Roberti, on a plane, and they began discussing a plan that Smokey had developed for a juice powder that he was calling Juice on the Run. Smokey was very familiar with the juicing craze of the time because he had worked with "the Juiceman," Jay Kordich. From that experience, Smokey had come up with the idea to put juice powders in a capsule. I remember reading the summary of his business plan and thinking how unique this was as an idea and a product that could transform the juice craze and take it to the next level. I have never had a business plan excite me more in the twenty years I've been in business.

Jeff and I took the plan to a company in Memphis, Tennessee called National Safety Associates (NSA). NSA had a long history of successful marketing ventures including smoke detectors, water filters, and air filters. The founder of NSA, Jay Martin, is one of those inimitable entrepreneurs who has a keen sense about unique products and recognizes emerging trends before everyone else does. We knew a partnership with Smokey, Jay, and NSA would change the world, especially with the talented team Jay had at his company. From this partnership came a product called Juice Plus+®.

Juice Plus+® is now the most researched—and most widely sold—nutraceutical in history. Eleven independent studies on the product have been published, and NSA has achieved over $2 billion in sales in twenty-seven countries. Looking back fifteen years, I don't think it is even possible to measure the contribution Juice Plus+® has made to the well-being of countless people around the world. I have sat in conferences and listened to so many testimonials on how Juice Plus+® has changed people's lives. In the end, I think the impact of this product defines the real value of Juice Plus+® and Smokey Santillo.

In typical Smokey fashion, Juice Plus+® was not the end of his work but instead the impetus to contribute at an even higher level. While many people would have taken the money they made on such a venture and cut back on their efforts, Smokey says his success is a responsibility to elevate his ability to make a difference. NSA gave him a platform to develop additional products and educate millions on the value of whole-food nutrition. Every day Smokey continues to stretch the boundaries of alternative medicine with the sole focus of making a bigger difference in lives around the world. Ironically, some of his biggest fans used to be his biggest critics—the traditional medical practitioners. Smokey has predicted that healthcare in our society would move increasingly toward prevention and alternative medicine; contributing to this movement is at the forefront of his passion these days.

For those of you about to embark on reading Smokey's newest book, *ProMetabolics*, I offer the following advice: pay close attention to what he is telling you. Smokey's gifts ultimately benefit those who utilize them.

While some of his ideas and concepts might seem "outside the box," they are the future in Smokey's eyes. The theories, information, and methods he outlines in this book are at the forefront of alternative medicine. ***ProMetabolics* is every person's guide to achieving the best possible function of the human machine.** Although so much of the information we are given today is driven by personal or commercial agendas, Smokey is an exception to that rule. He writes and teaches for the sole purpose of positive change. Given his past success, I suspect this current venture—*ProMetabolics*—will be the next enlightening chapter in Smokey's quest to change the face of medicine and health in our world.

Gordon D. Hester
Finance and Business Management
The Roberti Companies
www.Roberti.net

PURPOSE OF THIS BOOK

"Every problem carries the seed of an equivalent or greater benefit."

My background is in nutrition, philosophy, and metaphysics. When I first sat down to write this book, I didn't think much about the philosophical angle; I just wanted to express some of the truths I had learned about nutrition. I have been blessed with great teachers who have guided me, and I've always received the proper answers when I needed them. As questions arise about specific aspects of nutrition, a book or another teacher appears. We all find ourselves in the position of looking for answers, for something that will make life easier or at least more understandable. Questions keep coming up: Why did this happen to me? Or, how did I get myself in this situation?

Every situation is a guided question to a hidden prayer. I believe that no matter what we're confronted with, it is a gift, and if we persevere, the right answer will come—unless we already know what the answer is and have chosen not to listen. Disease is no different. We attract it and bring it to ourselves in most situations. Consciously or unconsciously, we create it; it is unique to us and we own it. To find such truths is sometimes very difficult—but if it were easy, it would not be worth it.

If you're reading this book, you are a health seeker. You're someone who wants the best out of life, and you've been digging through books, maybe even attending seminars, trying to figure out the right diet for you. Or, you have an illness and you're trying to help yourself get well. In either case, you will surely find the health answers you're seeking, and I pray that this book will help you in some small way.

The truth is sometimes hidden. In our quest, we seek, then we find, and we realize that the truth was there all the time. Our individual paths are so special and unique. If we look at everything in life as being significant to us, then our path will become clear. "Small is the gate and narrow the path to life, and only a few find it" (Matt. 7—HS). Throughout most of our lives, we are convinced or blinded through propaganda, special interest groups, or professionals who just don't know; but there is always someone with the answers. Thousands of years ago, the truth was known by great healers, and today these truths are resurfacing.

Disease is a process. It starts somewhere in our bodies and spreads from there; if we want to heal it, we have to approach it from within. The symptoms we experience when we're sick are just a cover, a blanket that is not telling us what the core of our problem really is. All symptoms are manifestations of the body's attempt to rebalance itself. Not only is disease a process, but your own disease is unique to you. Treatment, whether drug therapy, nutritional therapy, or something else, is therefore not a one-size-fits-all proposition. Not everyone who shares similar symptoms needs the same vitamins or medications.

Many theories out there propose systems to determine the type of foods or therapies you need. Some systems point you in the direction of foods and supplements chosen according to identifiable, unchanging features of your body's inherent constitution such as your metabolic type or blood type. I've learned so much from reading about these systems. But we are emotional beings, we get ill, we exercise, we undergo various new experiences all the time, and any of these things can change our chemistry. This can mean that on a daily basis we have changing nutritional needs— so knowing your metabolic type and your blood type is not enough.

The monitoring system in this book identifies metabolic changes you are going through so you may determine at any given point in time what you need nutritionally. You change daily. If you're angry, or eating a lot of carbohydrates, or experience something tragic, these events and factors can immediately acidify your body, and you need to know what to do. They can change you for quite a while if they're unaddressed and allowed to continue. The monitoring system gives you an instant answer about what to do. You may be a laid-back person, but various stressors can tax your nervous system, drive up your adrenal glands' activity, burn your sugars more rapidly, and push your thyroid gland to the limit regardless of your "normal" constitution. Fortunately, with the self-monitoring protocol in these pages, you will be able to recognize what's going on, adjust quickly, and bring yourself back to your balanced state.

Every situation, every meal, every emotion is personal to you, and balancing your chemistry is personal as well. I like to call it "balancing your terrain." The great philosopher, Popeye, said, "I am what I am." You are what you are at any given moment, and it's good to know this because disease is a process, and every day you experience various emotions and situations that can push you away from your natural state of health.

Using my monitoring system is like telling the future. For example, I deal with many high school and college athletes in my practice, and in monitoring them over the years, I've noticed that some have developed an iodine deficiency. This lowers their thyroid activity. It doesn't matter what blood type or constitution they might have—they have become tired, irritable, and overly acidic. When this happens, their supplements and diet need to be changed immediately, because even though they might perform well and look good for now, the process taking place is heading toward rapid aging and disease.

If you have allergies, Candida, autoimmune disease, fibromyalgia, or arthritis, these conditions fluctuate all the time. By monitoring the changes in your digestive system and the pH of your saliva, urine, blood, and other tissues, you can turn any of these disease processes around. Or, if you want to fast for any particular health purpose and your saliva turns acidic, the suggestions in this book will make for an easier fasting process. The chapters about fats, phytochemicals, insulin, enzymes, nutrition, and more are packed full of useful information. Coupled with the monitoring system, they will give you a personalized, specific direction to take toward a healthful balance.

Twenty-five years of clinical experience using every diet imaginable, training athletes of all ages, and working with over 20,000 clients made me realize that we all need a system, a simple and inexpensive system that we can use at home to monitor our bodies and the changes we experience. We need a system to guide us in our choice of foods and supplements and give us a way to help ourselves when we're sick or in a crisis. This book presents a monitoring system that I, and many of my clients, have found to be very successful.

Please note: no criticism of any other dietary theory is implied. Many of these theories are excellent and have their place. The do-it-yourself, at-home monitoring system in this book will not conflict with whatever you are presently doing, but only add to it. It can even be used to monitor your current treatment strategy or nutritional regimen, if any. It can be applied in various situations; you can monitor your body's response to a food, a crisis, a fever, a cold or flu, a supplement, a fast, or a detoxification regime. I hope my system helps you and adds to the knowledge and wisdom you already possess.

INTRODUCTION: WHAT YOU WILL LEARN

"Know the truth, and the truth will set you free."

This book is based on my twenty-five years of experience in the healing arts. I've counseled over 20,000 clients and continually find that at all times, the whole body must be balanced for optimal health to be achieved. Whether the problem is a common cold or cancer, the body must be brought back to its normal balance, called homeostasis. There are many ways to do this; the problem is selecting which to use. Once you understand *the true cause of disease*, it is much easier to choose the method or therapy you need.

Keep in mind that an underlying health issue can have some surprising effects because of the interconnectedness of the body's tissues, organs, and systems. You may feel a pain in your shoulder that was actually caused by a gall bladder problem or some other focus of infection remote from the pain. A tooth infection can become an infection throughout your body, causing joint pain for years without the source being detected. You will learn in the first part of this book that symptoms are only an indication that something is wrong, and not necessarily at the symptoms' location.

You will also learn that when we call something a genetic condition, we're often really saying, "We just don't understand." As Jeffrey Bland states in his wonderfully written book, *Genetic Nutritioneering*: "Your genes alone are not responsible for your health. Instead, your health depends principally on the way you influence the expression of your genes throughout the collective experience of your life." *(Bland JS, Benum SH. Genetic Nutritioneering. Keats Publishing, New Canaan, CT, 1999.)* He demonstrates throughout his book that virtually thousands of substances in foods can either promote or suppress the specific activities or expressions of genes. Health or disease can therefore be promoted by the food we eat, because it creates the environment that our cells live in. This gives you a tremendous amount of freedom, because it means that if your parents or grandparents died of a certain disease, you don't necessarily have to die of the same disease. We have certain hereditary tendencies—strengths or weaknesses—but we now know that we can control these tendencies through diet and lifestyle choices.

If your father has heart problems and you eat a high-starch diet, use toxic fats, don't exercise, and smoke, then what would you expect to result? The same condition your father has. Now I ask you: is that genetics? Very few genetic diseases are caused solely by faulty genes; most can be "resisted" by a healthy lifestyle, especially by good nutrition. If you trace your ancestry through several generations, you'll probably find that the diseases now prominent in your family tree didn't even exist back then. This book will teach you what brought them into present generations, and you will have the opportunity to eliminate those diseases from your own life. They may have something to do with the 70,000 chemicals in our modern environment—what do you think?

I have faced two major illnesses in my lifetime. Neither one exists in my body any longer. Through knowledge and understanding, I eliminated both conditions. Knowledge is the greatest tool. Although we've been taught to believe that the symptom is the problem, this is far from the truth. The truth is that the body's terrain—its fluids and tissues—becomes toxic at the site of infection. These toxins can cause scarring and inflammation. These local disturbances, in turn, can radiate from the original focal point to far-distant places by way of the nervous system, energy meridians, and bloodstream. This distribution of an infection or its effects throughout the body is known as the causal chain. (Don't get discouraged if you encounter some unfamiliar terms; I promise I'll make things simple and clear as you travel through this book.)

As an example, let's say you have a sinus infection. It produces fluid and phlegm that drains into your stomach and intestines, causing bloating, gas, stomach upset, burning urine, headache, diarrhea, weakness, fever, and tremendous fatigue. Which symptoms are you going to treat? The best answer is none of them in particular, and all of them in general. The main focus of infection may be the sinuses, but through the process of disease and your body's efforts to rebalance, many symptoms are being presented. This can confuse doctors who don't understand the *true* cause of disease, and they may treat only your stomach or your diarrhea without recognizing the focus of infection.

And all diseases are like this. They produce one or more symptoms, sometimes a whole cascade of symptoms, even those as intangible as emotional anxiety, fear, or simply being unpleasant and feeling uncomfortable. If you try to suppress your symptoms by using the wrong nutritional supplements or drugs, you drive the symptoms and poisons deeper into the body, only for them to express themselves again, or differently, later on. If suppressed yet again, they can develop into chronic disease. From this book, you will learn that you can help the body heal itself by *changing the process of disease.*

Symptoms are merely pictures that lie on top of the process. You wouldn't treat a diseased tree by painting its browning leaves green, would you? You shouldn't approach your own symptoms that way either. You must change the process of disease by changing your body's terrain. "Terrain" in this case simply means blood, urine, saliva, glandular secretions, and connective tissue, and I'm going to add the endocrine system to those because it controls hormonal secretions. The terrain can be considered as the environment that your cells live in. This book presents a system of balancing your body's terrain by monitoring and adjusting the pH of your urine and saliva, your body temperature, and your blood pressure. By following this simple system, you will be able to observe what your diet and supplements are (or are not) doing for your body. You will also be able to speed your recovery from illnesses and injuries, lose weight naturally, monitor your detoxification program, balance your thyroid and adrenal glands' activity, and personalize your diet to include the foods and supplemental nutrients that best suit you.

I've always said that the doctor of the future will be one who tells his patients what type of doctor to go to. What type of doctor should you go to when you're confused about what your symptoms mean? If a shoulder pain can be caused by a gall bladder problem, how do you know who to see for diagnosis and treatment? This book will help you figure that out. By reading it, you'll gain such a tremendous amount of knowledge about disease that what you have to do to change the process of disease by bringing the body back to its healthy state will become apparent—or at the very least, your new understanding will point you in the right direction, to the right type of doctor. A physician who knows several types of therapies can better detect complicated pathologies and their causal chains.

Please relax and take your time reading—don't skip chapters. This book has been called the story of truth by many. Stay well.

– Dr. Humbart "Smokey" Santillo

PART ONE

The Cause of Disease

DISEASE IS NOT ITS SYMPTOMS

As I mentioned in the Introduction, symptoms are only the clothing of a disease process. Although the same symptoms can appear in many people, their causes can be quite different. At first when you read this chapter, you're going to ask yourself, "How can I find the cause of my symptoms if the symptoms are not the disease?" The answer will become apparent as you read on; at the very least, you'll know what type of doctor to seek.

The majority of human ailments are linked to diet and lifestyle. But we don't always want to admit this, for two reasons. First, it seems almost too simplistic. After all, how can eating food reverse disease and the aging process? (I'll show you.) Second, we just don't want to change what is comfortable. Some of us are not used to putting more than the slightest effort into our health. Taking a pill seems so much easier than paying attention. But your health is your responsibility, and diet and lifestyle awareness is the key to improving your health, so go for it.

The main objective at this point is to realize that we are all different genetically and biochemically, and that because of this fact, treatments can not be standardized. The one-size-fits-all approach to drugs and nutritional supplementation just isn't working. Compare your body to a car: some cars run on diesel, some on high-test, and some on regular—they don't all require the same fuel, and neither do we.

Your dietary needs are based on genetic predispositions, blood type, metabolic characteristics, geographical location, and how your immune system is adapting to whatever is going on in your life at the present time. If an illness is present, your diet has to be regulated accordingly. We can easily see how different we are from each other on the surface, in such things as our hair, skin, fingerprints, and bone structure, so it shouldn't be hard to fathom that we are also different below the surface. Within our genetic melting pot, you are an individual at all levels of your being.

Modern pharmaceutical science with its mass-market approach is not the solution to modern lifestyle-based illness. For instance, a single type of drug, usually whatever remedy is currently trendy, is prescribed to most asthmatics. The same approach is often taken with nutritional remedies, but using the same herb for all asthmatics isn't the answer either. Of course, you can't blame nutrition experts for wanting to duplicate the same results with the same formulas on similar health problems, or for wanting a single diet or a particular herbal formula to optimize everybody's health. But as I have learned, it doesn't work that way.

This disappointment led me to a deeper understanding of disease. In a heterogeneous society like ours, things just aren't that easy! Maybe I shouldn't say this—maybe I should say, "We have to change our approach." Once I understood disease as a process and understood that the treatment approach has to be individualized, it opened up a new world to me.

With all of our society's wealth, scientific advancement, and investment in pharmaceutical research, why are Americans the unhealthiest people in the world? In the last fifteen years, obesity has risen 32 percent (25 percent in children), and 40 percent of current applicants for service in the U.S. Armed Forces are rejected because of poor health. Don't get me wrong—I love seeing what's going on in the sciences and how research in both mainstream and alternative medicine is bringing different schools of thought together in the attempt to solve our health problems. If that weren't happening, I wouldn't be able to write this book. I see the value in both pharmaceutical and nutritional science—why pick sides? After all, if I get hit by a car and my guts are lying on the street, please don't take me to an herbalist. Health research is an evolutionary, necessary process, and the fact remains, as ever, that no one person or side has all the answers.

Let me use an example of a hormone imbalance to give you an idea of what I mean by disease being a process. Whenever you eat starch or sugar (carbohydrates), your blood sugar level rises, and your pancreas responds by pumping the hormone insulin into your bloodstream to drive that blood sugar (glucose) into your cells. Insulin does many necessary things in the body, but a high insulin level sets off a problematic causal chain. It activates cells throughout your body to absorb sugar, fats, and proteins. It influences your kidneys to hold on to salt and water. It narrows your arteries by stimulating the growth of smooth muscle cells in their walls and stimulating the growth of fibrous connective tissue that gives structure to the earliest-forming plaque deposits. And it drives your kidneys to flush out magnesium and potassium in your urine, which, in time, can lead to abnormal, even deadly heart rhythms such as fibrillation.

Let's take a look at a confusing group of symptoms covering up an imbalance in just one hormone. Insulin goes up because of one main factor, and that's diet: specifically, eating a diet high in sugar and refined grains day after day. The most common symptom of too much insulin is adult-onset, or type II, diabetes. But there's actually much more to this disease process. When your blood sugar and insulin levels rise, your body stores unused glucose as glycogen and as fat—so you get fatter. The loss of magnesium and potassium through your kidneys increases the acidity of your blood, which can cause fatigue, headaches, diarrhea, skin conditions, and heart irregularities. Your thickened arterial walls lead to arteriosclerosis and heart disease. Because of your narrowing vessels and your kidneys' extra water retention, you now have high blood pressure.

Which problem do you treat first? All of these symptoms are on the surface of high insulin secretion. Is injecting more insulin the answer? Or should we trace the condition back to the diet that is upsetting the body's biochemistry and stimulating high insulin secretions to begin with?

The longer you have a condition, the farther it reaches within the body, causing other complications. What was once acute becomes chronic. You can't cure the whole thing at once. Time will heal, but the body's healing process follows its own priorities—first things first, last things last. For example, if you have irritable bowel symptoms, your elimination of toxins is slower than usual, so these poisons build up, causing a sinus infection and an ear-ache. This makes sense when you remember that the bloodstream touches every cell in your body within a few minutes. The body then tries to balance itself through detoxification by way of elimination, first through cleaning out the intestinal tract; then, once toxin build-up is eliminated, the sinus and ear-ache clear up on their own.

Let's go back to the insulin experience. As described, a high-carbohydrate diet can cause high blood pressure, heart disease, arteriosclerosis, and kidney problems. This whole process is signaling that something is wrong by demonstrating this variety of symptoms. Now you can understand that these symptoms are part of a disease process and that each symptom can't possibly be the disease itself. *Change the process, and you change the surface expression of symptoms.* Things only look complicated—they could actually be very simple. Healing disease by changing the process is like peeling an onion. Layer by layer, the body keeps healing until it gets to the core problem. Then the final healing takes place and you become symptom-free.

By using the system in this book to monitor and balance your internal terrain, you will see exactly how your body is handling whatever state or condition you are experiencing. This check-and-balance system will show you what your lifestyle, stress level, and diet are doing to you—and that enables you to change your direction by monitoring your supplements and your diet. In other words, you can change the process from sickness to health, from disease to healing, and maintain a healthy balance.

THE FOCUS AND DEVELOPMENTAL PROCESS OF DISEASE

Disease always has to start somewhere. Knowing that symptoms are just the outer expression of a process that had a specific beginning, common sense tells us that we have to get to the cause of the symptoms. This is called finding the focus (or, if there is more than one, the foci).

The focus is usually a segment of infected tissue from which disease-causing bacteria, viruses, and their toxins spread through the blood and lymph and circulate to other parts of the body. Usually they deposit themselves or establish headquarters in weak areas in our bodies, where they produce another symptom far from the original source. This area is called a field of disturbance. "Field of disturbance" and "symptom" are synonymous terms. You can have one focus and many symptoms.

A focus can be an infected tooth, tonsils, adenoids, old scars, or an intestinal infection. It can be heavy metal or drug accumulation, emotional stress, or a surgery. A focus can be an area of the body that's chronically inflamed or under constant insult, such as lungs subjected to smoking or joints injured through ongoing improper exercise. For instance, I've seen heavyweight lifters who weigh 350 pounds and are squatting 600–700 pounds; their knees wear out, causing inflammation and bacterial infections. Basically, a focus is any place in the body where disease begins.

Because the primary cause of a focus is a changed internal environment, treating the secondary bacterial invasion with an antibiotic can't result in complete healing. In other words, such a treatment would attack a symptom that resulted from the disease process but not the cause of the disease. Any time you change the environment of your internal organs and tissues, you set the stage for infections and an immune system response, and you also disturb the function of the body's systems. For example, let's say you have too much caffeine, which irritates the nervous system, which stimulates the release of stored sugar, which stimulates the pancreas to secrete insulin, and so on—I could continue with this chain reaction, but I'm sure you get the point. The disturbances become more prominent as they continue over time and as the body's energy declines.

But at this point there are no morphological changes yet; that is, no apparent changes in physical structure or form. Something—maybe something you're doing—is irritating to the body. You feel uneasy, and you're experiencing sub-clinical symptoms such as fatigue, irritability, insomnia, difficulty concentrating, bowel irregularities, bloating, bad breath, and the like. When you report these symptoms to your doctor, he or she checks you out with traditional methods and says, "You're fine." If you're even asked, "Are you eating properly?" you could say yes or no, but either way, that's usually as far as it goes. Nothing really shows, so you're told to just keep on keeping on.

The change or irritation hasn't produced a focus yet, thus no direct diagnosis can be made—at least through traditional methods. But those of us who work with energy medicine know better. Sub-clinical symptoms eventually lead up to a clinically recognizable disease. Yet those disturbances are seldom diagnosed properly, because traditional tests don't reveal them. Functional disturbances can occur in both the emotional and physical fields of experience. For example, if you're depressed, your digestion will be slow, causing constipation and fatigue. Those are functional disturbances, but they wouldn't be clinically classified as disease. There is no morphological change, so the root problem remains "out of sight" from the perspective of many clinicians.

Functional medicine analyzes the disharmonies in systems and organs that precede acute and chronic disease. Functional disorders are those disharmonies, from which clinical ailments develop. Pathology is the study of the nature of disease and the structure and functional changes produced by disease. Doesn't it seem funny to study the "path of disease" but only treat the end symptoms?

Many physicians don't really understand that once a functional change begins, so has a disease. The cause is always at a place on the path before functional changes occur. Some physicians do try to identify and treat functional disturbances. Functional medicine embraces diagnostic methods that analyze the totality of the body's regulatory functions—its biophysical, biochemical, enzymatic, endocrine, immunological, and bioenergetic regulatory capacities.

To recap: The focus of a disease is established by an initiating cause—such as poor diet, smoking, or damage from free radicals—producing functional problems (undiagnosed) and sub-clinical symptoms, which eventually lead to a recognized, categorized diagnosis. The combination of the specific initiating irritant, its affinity for a particular system or organ in the body, and the person's genetic weaknesses will finally determine the resulting illness, which is an expression of that person's genetic and biochemical individuality.

In Summary

Therefore, to treat an individual's disease, we must find its focus (or foci) and identify the preliminary factors that led to the condition. We must eliminate the cause, treat the major focus, and maybe treat some of the most uncomfortable, prominent symptoms—as opposed to treating symptoms far away from the cause and even farther from the cure.

Most of us know what we're doing that's causing our fatigue and other sub-clinical disturbances. To treat yourself, you have to listen to your body and eliminate possible causes—in other words, "Be your own doctor." Remember that a focus can be at any bodily site and can produce a variety of symptoms. Toxins, viruses, and bacteria travel through the body and take hold of the weakened tissue sites, setting up another focus if left unmanaged for long periods of time.

Beware of the use of drugs in your treatment. Use them with caution and only when necessary. Know the side effects of anything you're taking, so there will be no surprises. Get off of them as soon as possible. Most importantly, don't use a drug to treat the side effect of another drug. Be aware of the effects you experience with any drug or other treatment, and be aware of your body's efforts to heal itself. Remember, as disease is a process, so is cure. While your body works to get rid of all the accumulated waste built up over the years, you may get a replay of some of your past ailments, but they'll pass. Keep this possibility in mind so as not to lose confidence in the natural process of healing.

Not only can using my self-monitoring system help you find the focus of your ailment, but it can also help you balance your body's terrain in order to address your sub-clinical symptoms. You'll be able to determine which organs are weak, which glands are out of balance, and which foods you should eat to redirect your pH and endocrine function. You'll learn to give your body what it needs and let it heal itself. You are programmed for health; you simply have to eliminate what is hindering your body's functions and give it the raw materials it needs.

WE ARE ALL SNOWFLAKES

L et's take a closer look at how unique you really are, and why disease is specific to each individual, and why drug or nutritional therapy for any disease should be tailor-made for the individual.

Dr. Roger Williams' book *Biochemical Individuality*, first published in 1956, presented what I consider to be a timeless message. *(Williams RJ. Biochemical Individuality. McGraw-Hill, New York, NY, 1998.)* He first gained recognition for showing that even identical twins could have different needs for their own optimal function. Although such twins share identical genes, their differing nutrition and developmental environments can result in different expression of those genes as they get older.

Dr. Williams' research demonstrated that we are not only different on the outside, but that our internal environment of organs, blood, tissues, and secretions are different from person to person. For example, he found that the amount of the enzyme pepsin in the gastric (stomach) juices varied at least a thousand-fold among a group of normal adults. When he studied the contents of blood, he found that its nutritional and chemical variations were vast, not only in adults but also in children. Basically, he demonstrated that virtually everything about us is unique.

From these facts, it is logical to propose that drugs and other nutritional substances can act differently within different people. An example of this is drug side effects. These are usually presented as a standard list for any given medication, but ten people taking the same drug can experience ten different side effects. Then when an additional drug is taken for those side effects, things really get complicated.

If you look at the figure below in the *Atlas of Human Anatomy*, you'll see nineteen very different-looking stomachs. *(Netter FH. Atlas of Human Anatomy, 4th ed. Saunders-Elsevier, Philadelphia, PA, 2006.)*

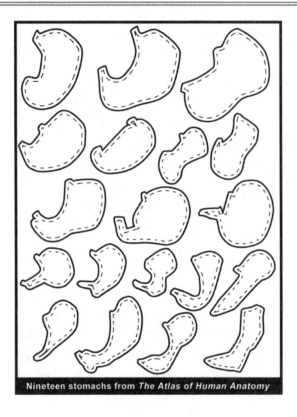

Nineteen stomachs from *The Atlas of Human Anatomy*

Just as the size of this organ (and others) can differ from person to person, so can secretions of hormones, digestive acids, and enzymes. Age-related enzyme decreases, for example, can significantly affect your digestion. Changes in enzyme levels are far-reaching when it comes to maintaining health or treating disease. If food is not digested properly, nutrient deficiencies result, which in turn affect hormonal levels, immunity, and the ability to repair normal cellular breakdown—this is called aging rapidly. Certain substances such as coffee and alcohol also destroy digestive enzymes. A holistic physician has to consider not only the variations in individuals but also what foods, drugs, and other things they're taking in or doing that can damage their organs and systems.

The genetic structure is no longer viewed as rigidly as it was previously. Scientists Jerry Bishop and Michael Waldholz make the following statement in their book, *Genome*: "Aberrant genes do not, in and of themselves, cause disease. By and large, their impact on an individual's health is minimal until the person is plunged into a harmful environment." *(Bishop JE, Waldholz M. Genome. Simon and Schuster, New York, 1990.)* In this context, "environment" means both the internal environment—the body's terrain, as described earlier—and the external exposure to chemicals and pollution.

It is now well recognized that the full set of genes you were born with, called the genotype, gets transformed into your phenotype, which is the result of gene expression and function after your genes have been influenced by nutrition, lifestyle, and other environmental factors. Therefore, genes alone do not give rise to disease.

In *Genetic Nutritioneering*, nutritionist Jeffrey Bland states, "Disease in most cases results when the individual elects a lifestyle or diet that alters the expression of the genes in such a way that the weakness or uniqueness of inheritance factors results in a phenotype we call disease." *(Bland JS, Benum SH. Genetic Nutritioneering. Keats Publishing, New Canaan, CT, 1999.)* Again, the phenotype is the result of your genes' expression after they have been influenced. The influence can, of course, be in a healthy direction instead of toward an unhealthy state. We have more power over disease than we thought. This puts the control back in your hands.

Williams pointed out that hair growth, healing time after surgery, weight gain, and sleep time after surgery can all be influenced by nutritional influences on gene expression. What I'm emphasizing at this point is that we are all different on all levels, and that disease and its symptoms are indigenous to the individual. Also, although we have inherent genetic tendencies, or strengths and weaknesses, their expression can be influenced in a healthy direction to avoid disease.

In most contemporary clinical situations, people are found to fit into personally unique biochemical profiles according to their genetic structure, nutritional status, and environment. Because of this, the validity of the U.S. Recommended Dietary Allowances (RDAs), developed by the Food and Nutrition Board of the National Research Council, is questionable. The human nutritional needs represented by the RDAs are based on the "average individual"—but there is no such person.

Most of us learned in our school days about Gregor Mendel, who developed the concept that dominant and recessive genetic characteristics were locked in stone. We're now proving, however, that the expression of genes can be modified through changes in diet and lifestyle. Williams coined the phrase "genotrophic disease" to describe diseases that result when genetically determined nutritional or metabolic needs are not being met, leading to poor gene expression in the individual.

Logically, we understand that the growth of a tree can be duplicated by planting its seeds in a good, healthy soil. But if you take healthy seeds from a full-grown tree and put them in soil that has nutrient deficiencies and fungus, you get an altered expression. We have all heard of gross abnormalities in human embryos as a result of particular nutritional deficiencies or the effects of certain chemicals. In this vein, Williams discusses experiments done on spores, which are a type of unicellular organism. Irradiating some spores produced mutants incapable of carrying out their normal chemical reactions. It was assumed that the radiation-caused mutations were permanent lesions. But when this assumption was tested by giving the mutants supplemental biotin, a B-vitamin, most of them resumed normal activity; others resumed normalcy when given the B-vitamin riboflavin. This showed how vitamins can influence gene expression even after irradiation damage.

When the researchers took the experiment further, they found that the mutant spores still had an inherent ability to resume normalcy; when grown at a lower temperature, the spores produced riboflavin on their own and grow normally. The important principle to be derived from these studies is the principle of total genetic memory: that is, an organism's genes can be diverted by "genetic blocks" from their normal expressions, but the organism still can maintain its inherent potentialities.

In another example of genetic memory, Dr. Ian Wilmet used a fully mature cell from the udder of an adult female sheep and cloned the now-famous lamb named Dolly. The fact that a lamb was produced from a single cell of a mature ewe shows that the genetic material was not changed during that original sheep's aging process. As Bland states, "Under the right conditions all the genetic information encoded as your inheritance—from every stage of development from an embryo to an elderly adult and from every cell type in your body—is potentially accessible to any cell on your body." This concept opens the door to the exciting theory that at any age you might access information encoded on your genes that can recreate a younger and healthier you.

Sickle cell anemia is an inherited condition in which the structure of hemoglobin, the iron-carrying red pigment in blood, is defective. The defective hemoglobin molecules stick to others and crystallize in the red blood cell, which then bends into a sickle shape. When this sickle cell travels through the bloodstream, it cuts the tissues it touches, causing severe pain. Forty-five years ago, Dr. Pawling Itano predicted that the disease of sickle cell anemia would someday be modified by changing the faulty gene's expression. *(Itano PL. Sickle cell anemia: a molecular disease. Science 1949 110:543-547.)* And in 1994, researchers found substances that, if administered to individuals who carried the sickle cell gene, changed its genetic expression. Butyrate, a salt contained in a fatty acid found in butter, is one of these substances. When a group of people with sickle cell anemia were given butyrate, they began to produce normal hemoglobin rather than the defective form—another demonstration that nutritional intervention can modify gene expression. Remember, your genes don't change, but their expression can indeed be changed.

It is a known fact that many drugs can change gene expression; this is why we experience side effects. Xanax is an anti-anxiety drug used to treat anxiety and panic disorders. According to the 2007 *Physicians' Desk Reference*, the side effects of Xanax are: outbursts of anger, depression, difficulty concentrating, behavioral problems, hallucinations, low blood pressure (causing fainting or confusion), rashes, memory impairment, muscle weakness, chills, sore throat and fever, ulcers (sores) of the mouth, yellowish tinge to skin, bruising, and bleeding. *(Physicians' Desk Reference 2007. Thomson PDR, Montvale, NJ, 2006.)*

Pretend you're a doctor whose patient has anxiety and is having panic attacks, so you prescribe Xanax. But you also have some knowledge of nutrition, so you have your patient get an amino acid analysis for a protein or amino acid deficiency, and the test indicates a deficiency in the amino acid tryptophan. Tryptophan happens to be responsible for the production of serotonin, which is a neurotransmitter that relaxes the brain, body, and nervous system. So as the good and loving doctor that you are, you prescribe tryptophan. Your patient's serotonin level then increases over a period of time and Xanax is no longer needed, because you found and addressed the cause of the problem.

The other treatment scenario would be to prescribe Xanax, look no further, and when the patient comes back with some of the side effects mentioned for Xanax, to prescribe another drug for the side effects. But that's getting further away from the cause and creating complications. If this patient then consults a nutritionally oriented doctor, that doctor might say, "I found that you have a problem digesting protein, and as a result, your tryptophan level is low and, consequently, so is your serotonin level. But before we can fix these problems, we have to support your system nutritionally, wean you off the Xanax, and then detoxify your system to clean out the drug residue, which will eliminate the drug's side effects and begin to correct your digestion." This approach is more like peeling the layers of an onion, which I mentioned in my earlier discussion of the natural healing process.

Many things have to be done before we get to the major focus of the problem. All of this hypothetical patient's symptoms can be seen as expressions of genetic variations determined by his or her heredity. The whole condition started with a digestive disturbance, which led to a biochemical and hormonal imbalance, which produced distinct symptoms because of genetics. Taking Xanax for some of those symptoms caused a group of other symptoms, all relative to the individual.

Let's say another patient comes in with those same symptoms of anxiety and panic attacks, and you prescribe the same therapy (temporary Xanax, plus tryptophan supplements) but find that it doesn't work. Upon further analysis, a high level of accumulated mercury is found to be the cause of this patient's problem. Then a third patient comes in, with different complaints: chronic fatigue, difficulty sleeping, and poor digestion. Through testing, you find a tryptophan deficiency once again, but this time without the symptoms of anxiety or panic attacks—because this patient has an inherently strong nervous system.

Williams personally experienced a similar situation with morphine, which led to his discoveries. His doctor tried to put him to sleep with a shot of morphine, but the morphine had the opposite effect, and kept his mind racing uncontrollably. This uncharacteristic reaction to morphine prompted Williams' realization that the different effects from different medicines, as well as the different effects from different nutrients, are indicators of all the different ways that genes can express themselves. The only way to make sense of someone's seemingly complicated symptoms is to pay attention to the person as an individual and find the focus, the major cause of the problem.

In Summary

We are all individuals at all levels of expression, from fingerprints to cellular activities, from the size of our organs to the contents of their secretions. Even twins develop differently when exposed to different environments. This means that growth, nutritional needs, and a disease's reaction to nutrients and drugs are indigenous to the individual. And because our cells maintain perfect memory of their genetic potential through the individual's lifetime, the possibility of reversing sickness and even some of the aging process is within reach. It's almost mind-boggling to think about what we can do for our own health if we figure out exactly what foods we need to eat and understand how biochemically unique we really are. We can actually change the expression of our genes through lifestyle, nutrition, and the therapies we choose when we get ill.

Ten people can have the same symptoms, but there can be ten different causes for them. For example, in a group of people who all have asthma, one may have asthma from smoking, another from improper diet, another from drug-suppressed allergies, and so on. That is one of the main reasons why it is so important to have a self-monitoring system such as the one described in this book. You can learn to assess and rebalance your biochemistry no matter what the cause of imbalance may be. And with this system, you will be able to build an individualized diet and supplement program that fits you as an individual.

Disease is also an individual proposition. People who have similar symptoms do not always need, or benefit from, the same nutrients or drugs. If a therapy is incorrect for the person receiving it, the disease can be driven deeper into the body and cause further complications. Pharmaceutical treatment often creates this scenario. This brings us to the topic of the next chapter: understanding the focus and development of disease through the theory of pleomorphism.

PLEOMORPHISM: THE LOST SCIENCE OF DISEASE

I initially wanted to call this chapter "Back to the Future," because the theory it presents was postulated centuries ago. But instead of tracing back before 1800, I chose to start with the work of Antoine Béchamp (1816–1908). Before his time, scientists had much less technical equipment to help them prove their points, although they did it in their own way and, as it turned out, they were right. *Germs themselves do not cause disease*—and, yes, Louis Pasteur was wrong.

Pasteur and Monomorphism

In the nineteenth century, Pasteur's germ theory became the medical paradigm for the Western world. He proposed that the body is sterile and that germs from the air cause disease. This idea became ingrained in medical science, and thereafter the search was on to "find the pill that cures disease." But despite the ensuring centuries of research, degenerative diseases are increasing; diabetes is increasing at an alarming rate; infectious diseases are on the rise; and AIDS, herpes, Epstein-Barr virus, Candida (yeast) infections, environmental illnesses, chronic fatigue, allergies, chemical sensitivities, and fibromyalgia are the latest challenges. We must admit that no cure-all pill has been found and that what we are doing is not working.

Pasteur's germ theory stated:
1. Diseases arise from germs outside the body.
2. Germs must be guarded against.
3. Their shape and function are constant.
4. Every disease has a primary causative microorganism.
5. Disease can affect anybody at any time.

The germ theory has been called monomorphism, from the roots "mono" for one and "morph" for body or form. By this theory, each disease has one cause, and to fight disease, we must find the germ and then find the drug that will kill the germ. But if germs from the air are the source of disease, as Pasteur said, why do primitive peoples today show very little degenerative disease until we provide them with sugar and processed food and displace them from their native environments? Believing in the germ theory takes our power and control over disease away from us. We think if we get sick, we can simply take the magic pill. There's absolutely no sense of personal responsibility. It's giving up our God-given healing force within. Most people don't understand that aside from inhaling or drinking a poison or stepping on poison ivy, we create disease through improper diet, lifestyle, and stress.

Béchamp, Rosenow, and Pleomorphism

Pasteur's colleague Antoine Béchamp (1816–1908) presented the competing idea that the body is not sterile and that under certain conditions, micro-organisms can evolve from within. His idea was the basis for the theory of pleomorphism, meaning "many forms." Béchamp discovered what he called microzymas, which he described as tiny, living granules residing in the body. He found that, under certain conditions, the microzymas could evolve into bacteria or "more pathogenic or disease-causing forms, causing the breakdown of the cell structure of its host." He also found that they were indestructible, could ferment or putrefy, and are still found living after the host organism dies.

Of course, Pasteur tried to discredit his rival, but he knew Béchamp was right and on his deathbed, his parting words were, "The microbe (germ) is nothing, the terrain is everything." The body's terrain, in general terms, is the following: the blood and other fluids that surround the cells;

connective tissue; the mesenchyma cells, a meshwork of embryonic connective tissue from which vessels and connective tissues are formed; and the parenchyma cells, which are cells that form the essential or functional elements of the organs (such as the kidney's nephrons or the brain's neurons). I also like to include the endocrine system as part of the terrain. This concept of the body's terrain will be detailed further in upcoming chapters.

Béchamp's disease theory is:

1. Diseases arise within the body by the action or influence of living microorganisms (microzymas).
2. These microorganisms are usually healthy and even assist the body in normal immune functions.
3. These microorganisms can change shape, color, and even size (pleomorphism), according to the terrain.
4. If the body's terrain becomes toxic and less alkaline, these microorganisms can become pathogenic.

Symptoms are always evidence of the body trying to balance itself because of a changed environment. A person's several symptoms do not indicate several separate diseases. They are all different manifestations of the same root cause: an imbalanced, toxic terrain.

The pleomorphic life cycle of microbes was later demonstrated by Dr. Edward Rosenow, who was associated with the Mayo Clinic in the early 1900s and wrote over 450 papers on the cause of infectious diseases. He took several bacterial strains from various diseased tissues and placed them in separate Petri dishes containing a nutrient environment. After a short period of time, he examined them and found that they had all mutated into the same strain of bacteria. Then when he returned the mutated microbes back to the original diseased tissues, their offspring assumed the original forms and functions of the parent microbes. What this showed was that microorganisms change form depending on their environment, and that they can revert to the original form and produce offspring in that form when returned to their original environment. In other words, pleomorphism is when microbes show cyclic changes relative to their terrain.

Rife's Discovery

Dr. Royal Rife was a genius educated in the fields of optics, electronics, biology, and chemistry. He designed and built medical instruments including optical tools, spectroscopes, and stop-motion photomicrographs. The U.S. government and several other countries awarded him fourteen medals for his scientific achievements.

Dr. Rife built a number of microscopes that were far superior to any of his time and have never been duplicated. His most powerful, the Universal Microscope, was built in 1933, weighed 200 pounds, and had 5,682 parts. It stood 3 feet high and had a magnification of 31,000–60,000 diameters. Its optical system of numerous lenses and prisms included an illuminating unit with block crystal quartz prisms, through which the light would polarize (break up into definite patterns or vibrate in definite patterns) as it passed through, thereby illuminating the specimen for observation without killing it.

For studying microorganisms, this microscope was superior to the electron microscope, which requires that the specimen be stained with dye to be easily seen; the staining chemical kills the specimen, making it impossible to observe its life cycles or changes in form and function—its pleomorphism. When we examine a virus or bacteria with today's electron microscopes, we see only a snapshot of it at a particular stage of growth and we are fooled into thinking that what we've found is what causes the disease we're studying, when, in reality, the microorganism can change forms under different environmental or terrain conditions.

Developing a drug that destroys an organism during one stage of its cyclic development will only alter it (for example, in the case of bacteria or fungi, by destroying its outer membranes) at that stage of development, and also causes a chemical change in its environment, prompting it to adapt to and cycle into another form or level of growth: pleomorphism. Meanwhile, there is mounting evidence that drug-resistant microbes are gaining ground worldwide. Dr. Alexander Tomasz says, "We have been living in an era when if you got sick, there was always a pill to take. We are approaching an era when that will no longer be true." And he's right. Until we learn the true causes of disease (hint: not the germs) and take responsibility for our own health, this situation will continue, and worsen.

Rife discovered through observation that microbes change according to their environment. He concluded: "The body itself is chemical in nature which provides a certain medium which bacteria normally present feed on. These bacteria reproduce and are themselves composed of chemicals. Therefore, if the media upon which they feed becomes changed from the normal, it stands to reason that these same bacteria will also undergo a change chemically since they are feeding upon a media which is not normal to them. And that they pass through different stages of growth emerging to an entirely new entity similar to the morphological change as is the caterpillar to the butterfly... The majority of the viruses have been definitely revealed as living organisms, foreign substances it is true, but which once were normal inhabitants of the human body."

As an example of those "normal inhabitants," consider that we all have strep bacteria in our mouths, but you don't get strep throat until your mouth becomes acidic and the microbe changes, adapting to the change in terrain; then, its secretions, not the germ itself, cause strep throat. Similarly, if you're exposed to the flu virus, you'll only come down with a case of the flu if your blood is sufficiently toxic for the virus to take hold. That's why not everybody gets the flu when it's "going around."

Rife used different light frequencies to examine different microbes. A frequency, measured in the number of cycles per second, is the oscillation or "back and forth movement" of an energy emission—in this case, a wave of light energy. He realized that each microbe in each of its cycles of growth had specific corresponding frequencies. Everything, in fact, has a frequency at which it vibrates. Rife thought that if he could view a microbe with a certain light frequency, maybe he could kill it with the same frequency. And that's exactly what he did. This phenomenon is similar to when an opera singer hits a certain note and, across the room, a glass shatters because that specific note's frequency (as a wave of sound) matches what is called the resonant frequency of the glass.

As mentioned, Rife's microscope could illuminate the microbe of interest without killing it. He developed a Beam Ray, a tube with a cathode ray, which could emit frequencies equivalent to infrared radiation, ultraviolet radiation, x-rays, visible light rays, and radio waves. By matching the emitted frequency to the frequency of a specific microbe, the Beam Ray could be used to shatter them in a way similar to the glass phenomenon described above.

The problem with microscopes today is that a light shines through the bottom and up to the eyepiece. As the light travels up through the tube, the beams of light cross over each other within the tube. This limits the resolution or the ability to break up and separate the light; Rife realized better resolution was necessary to visualize and destroy microbes in the way he intended. In his microscope, the light did not cross.

In Rife's illuminating unit, when light passed from the light source through the block crystal quartz prisms, it was polarized, or divided into two beams that wouldn't cross. One beam was refracted off to the side of the prism, while the other beam passed through the prism to illuminate the specimen. Rotating the prism caused it to send specific beams within the light spectrum, from infrared through visible colors to ultraviolet, through the specimen as desired.

When the light frequency coming from the prism was in exact accord with the frequency of the organism or specimen Rife was examining, the specimen literally lit up, and he could observe the specimen by the light that was given off. As the light passed up through the specimen, he could observe its own true chemical color and its structure. Rife then developed a method to filter out any extra colors except the specific one he needed for a particular microbe. This is how he observed their growth cycles as they changed from a cell-deficient non-virulent form to a bacterium, virus, or fungus. (To view this phenomenon, go to www.VibrantHealth.com.)

But Rife wanted to cure disease, not just observe viruses and bacteria, so he developed the Beam Ray Tube. The tube was filled with gas that would emit various frequencies of light (visible, infrared, or ultraviolet) when light was passed through it, with which he intended to destroy particular microbes. He also figured out how to use high-frequency radio waves to transmit those specific frequencies toward the microbes. In other words, two levels of transmission would occur simultaneously: the "carrier" radio wave plus the "destroyer" light wave frequency that would kill the microbe of interest at whatever stage of its existence it could be found (virus, bacteria, and the like).

When Rife beamed the correct specific frequencies through the tube with a pulse-type activity, "on and off," the microbes he wanted to destroy would change color while absorbing the frequency, and they would die, sometimes shattering and disappearing. This is quite different from using an antibiotic to try to kill bacteria at just one stage of growth. Because each microbe can go through several different cycles of growth, you have to be able to recognize all of the different forms they can take, not just the one, in order to eliminate the microbe of interest. It is thought that there are hundreds of different strains of bacteria and viruses—it would be more correct, however, to recognize many configurations and activities at different growth cycles.

Rife's in-lab experiments soon found clinical application. In the 1930s, Beam Ray therapy was in use across America to destroy numerous pathogenic microorganisms like *Escherichia coli (E. coli)*, streptothrix, staphylococci, and typhus. People receiving this therapy were recovering from chronic ailments, with some of these cases well documented. In 1934, the University of Southern California Medical School verified the cases of sixteen different patients who'd been diagnosed as terminally ill but who showed no signs of cancer after thirty sessions with Rife. *(Lynes B. The Cancer Cure That Worked. Compcare Publications, Minneapolis, MN, 1987.)*

Enderlein and Endobiants

The work of Dr. Günther Enderlein (1872–1968) in a field known as biological medicine spanned more than sixty years. He identified small protein-like bodies in the blood, which he named endobiants, and noticed that these cell-wall-deficient proto-microbes exhibit more than one type of life cycle; he called this cyclogeny. He found that the primal endobiant lives symbiotically "in a mutually beneficial relationship" with the body's cells. The endobiant's life cycles include viral, bacterial, and fungal stages. As long as the body's pH stayed in its normal range, these endobiants live in harmony with the host, populating every part of the terrain.

Dr. Enderlein's endobiants are Béchamp's microzymas. Enderlein, like Béchamp, opposed Pasteur's theory that bacteria enter the body and produce disease. Using the technique of dark-field microscopy to examine live blood samples, Enderlein found that endobiants can evolve into higher and more active forms of expression. Dark-field microscopes with high magnification enable a nearly invisible microorganism to be visualized in front of a dark background with light being angled into the specimen from the sides. The light coming through the specimen is shifted into beams, one slightly out of phase with the other, called "phase contrast." Enderlein was able to deliver clear proof of the endobiant's ability to change from its original primal form all the way up to its cycle as a fungus. His studies revealed that the origin of disease is within.

While an endobiant is in its primal phase, it is beneficial to the body. If the terrain's pH becomes too acidic or too alkaline, the endobiant begins a growth cycle and becomes pathogenic, with the form it takes (bacterial, viral, or fungal) being relative to the terrain conditions. When and if the terrain's proper pH is restored, the more pathogenic forms cycle back down into the benign, symbiotic primal form, and its byproducts leave the body through the organs of elimination; but if the body cannot restore its balance, the endobiant progresses to a destructive, parasitic fungus form.

The important point here to remember is that once the terrain becomes normal again, a fungus or bacteria can devolve—that is, change back to its normal state. An example of this occurs in beer, to which yeast is added to begin the fermentation process; once the process is over and the terrain has changed, there is very little yeast left in the beer. Where did it go? It actually cycled back to its primal endobiant stage. This phenomenon can be observed under dark-field microscopes. And in the body, it is the only way healing can take place. We must bring our terrain back to normal pH.

As the endobiant grows in an acidic, toxic terrain, it becomes larger and secretes its own lactic acid and citric acid wastes, which are very toxic to the body. It poisons the terrain on an ongoing basis if not halted, until finally the endobiant cycles into a fungal, even cancerous condition. As Enderlein described, "Cancer is for the host organism a fermentation and decomposition condition, forced upon by a parasitic fungus and its developmental forms. These funguses devour protein, causing vascular changes, congestion, mucous elimination, arthritis, spondylosis, diabetes, tumors of all types, anemia, leukemia, and paralyses."

The first noticeable symptom of most diseases is a fever. Fever is the body trying to rid itself of the products of abnormal fermentation and decomposition, thereby clearing up the terrain and returning the endobiant to its original state. Pathogenic organisms cannot live beyond certain high temperatures, so the body cooks them and in the process gives you headaches, diarrheas, colds, flu, weakness, and fatigue. These symptoms are not separate diseases, but different manifestations of the same thing. The body uses all its eliminative organs—skin, eyes, ears, bowels, lungs, kidneys—to get rid of acidic wastes.

What triggers the primal endobiants' transformation from benign to pathogenic is that the body's terrain becomes acidic through poor diet and stress and toxicity. Cells under stress produce lactic and citric acid waste. In response, the cell-membrane-deficient endobiants gather together to form a more highly developed entity with a cell wall and nuclei, for protection from its changing environment. As these globular endobiant clusters begin to grow and cycle through their phases, they become aggressive toward the body. Certain conditions cause them to cycle into disease-causing forms including bacteria and viruses. If they continue to a fungal phase, the development of chronic diseases begins. The developed endobiant begins attacking and penetrating normal white blood cells, red blood cells, and more, breaking them down, which puts even more acid into the terrain. The body becomes over-acidic and congested.

As the body becomes acidic, congested, and full of byproducts of cellular debris and mucus, the blood's oxygen content decreases. If this process continues, our normal cells, instead of using oxygen to breathe aerobically, begin to convert to an anaerobic "fermentating type of cell" just to survive. This type of cell is a cancer cell, and it's trying to survive like every other cell in the body. We call it a cancer cell, but what it really represents is the power within: the cell is living at a disease level, which is a survival tactic of the body. As I've said, we are programmed to survive.

This process of the endobiant changing to a fungus is a normal process in response to the body getting toxic. The endobiant is trying to stay alive by breaking everything down until the host organism's death. Dead bodies, after all, are full of live fungus. During every stage of the disease process, the blood and tissues are releasing alkaline minerals such as calcium, potassium, sodium, iron, and magnesium bicarbonate into the body's terrain to neutralize the acids, but unfortunately this leads to developing mineral deficiencies and diseases such as osteoporosis and neurological disorders. The body is stealing from Peter to pay Paul. This is, however, another normal breaking-down process over which we have control and can, in some cases, reverse.

Physical or emotional stress, of course, is a factor in all disease. Under stress, your body's cells produce excess lactic acid, which adds to the fire or even triggers the disease process. At the beginning of this whole process, the body begins to experience functional disturbances not yet diagnosable by most medical means. When stress begins to build, symptoms not yet categorized as disease, such as depression, weakness, poor memory, sores, hoarseness, mucous, hearing loss, and vision loss, are just the beginning of a more serious manifestation. At this stage, if you are aware, you can easily remove the causal stressor, whether it's emotional conflict or a poor diet, and the body will return to its healthy state.

But if an infection presents itself and you do not use natural therapeutics to aid the body and instead use antibiotics, you add more wood to the fire. Antibiotics also produce an acidic effect on the body when they kill bacteria. In actuality, antibiotics destroy the bacterial wall, releasing protein matter and DNA fragments, creating pH changes in the body that enable surviving endobiants to start their infectious cycle all over again. This disturbance of the terrain is why infections can often get worse after treatment. A perfect example of this is the pharmaceutical treatment of a Candida infection, which "destroys" the yeast, but then the endobiants develop into a higher fungal form.

Most chemotherapeutic drugs in cancer treatment are anti-fungal. They destroy the fungus temporarily and the patient goes into remission. But in many cases, as we've all observed, the cancer comes back, and then when the same drug is used, it doesn't work any longer. Drugs become less effective as microbes have more of a virulent response to them. There is tremendous intelligence at all levels of existence.

You know that electrons and protons make up atoms, which make up molecules, and on upward through cells to organs and systems. Béchamp stated, "Microorganisms occur in diverse developmental stages and in diversified forms, from small rings of electrons up to large multi-nucleic organisms such as bacteria and fungus." If we look deeper into the causative factors of disease, we see that what changes at the top must change at the bottom, or what changes from the bottom must cause changes at the top. Simply put, when your terrain changes, your physics change too. The electrons and molecules that make up your cells begin a structural change of the cells. Along with this, your body's chemistry is changing. The terrain's pH is changing, cellular secretions are changing, and you become chemically imbalanced.

Taking drugs, which alter your chemistry even more, produces further chemical changes. Now it's the domino theory: for every cause there is an effect. Granted—and please remember that I said this—there is a place for the proper use of drugs. But they should always be monitored and complemented with natural therapeutics and a good diet. If you're working with a health-minded physician, it could be very possible to discontinue the use of drugs, balance your terrain, and bring your chemistry back to balance. I'm not against the use of drugs—I'm against the promiscuous use of them, and I'm against leaving people on them when it's not necessary. Each drug causes a chemical change in the body's terrain, either by inhibiting or stimulating other chemical changes.

Many of us have loved ones who sometimes take five or more drugs. Can you even imagine how far away from reality and balance they are? Anxiety and depression are terrible things. I was there during my battle with mercury poisoning. But I've been blessed with wonderful friends and family and healers who all chipped in and brought me back to normal. I was never left alone for two years. Someone was always by my side. Can you even imagine the love, security, and care I was receiving? I'm sure I was driving them all nuts, but they never gave up. Because of my experience, I've learned so much that I've been able, in turn, to help hundreds of other people and this book is the result of being inspired by my illness. Life is good.

Enderlein, through dark-field microscopy, was able to watch his endobiants evolve through all these stages. He developed isopathic therapy, which is the application of specific biological remedies for all of the non-specific general symptoms produced by the cyclic changes of disease conditions. His remedies help bring the body's terrain back to normal. Enderlein's isopathic formulas are a collection of harvested "spermit" endobiants at their simplest, non-virulent primal form. As these are taken into the body, they attack more highly developed, virulent endobiants in microbe form and break them back down to their normal primal "spermit" form. This is true healing.

I'm sure that more theories about pleomorphism and Enderlein's work will emerge, but they will only be improvements on what we already know to be true. (For more information on Enderlein's work, call 800-320-6036. For information on pleomorphism, see www.AntoineBechamp.com. For information on dark-field microscopes, see www.biomedx.com.)

I would like to thank Dr. Morris Zubkewych, my teacher, mentor, friend, and personal physician, for teaching me about pleomorphism. When I was ill, he monitored my healing process with his expertise in electral dermal screening and nutrition. When I first went to Dr. Zubkewych, I couldn't walk 100 yards, but he guaranteed me he'd have me up and running in no time. And that's exactly what I'm doing now. I'm back to training and have never felt better. If you're serious about getting well and want to take responsibility for your health, call Dr. Zubkewych's clinic (416-762-7591).

NUTRITION AND DISEASE

I thought you might find this material from an interview with Dr. D.J. Scott to be very enlightening. He is a personal friend and a long-time teacher of mine who has been practicing natural therapeutics—that is, treatment approaches including nutrition, herbs, fasting, and the like—for more than forty years. His approach is to get people well, no matter what it takes. I am deeply grateful for his contribution to this book.

Dr. Scott gives an interesting explanation of how our body's terrain becomes toxic and allows microorganisms to develop, and he puts the complexities of pleomorphism in easy-to-understand, layman's terms. He also discusses what has happened to our food supply over the last fifty years and how nutrient-deficient it has become. Years ago, food was nutrient-dense and could help us heal in a much more rapid fashion. But nowadays, the food generally available and eaten is not always our best medicine because of the ways it's grown and processed.

Dr. Scott poetically describes the healing force we have within and how the laws that apply within the body are the same laws that apply in our external environment. One of them, the law of selectivity, holds that at any particular time, a cell may need to take in something specific; another, the law of rejectivity, holds that a cell rejects what it does not need. Our bloodstream, the "river of life," should have everything our cells might need at the ready for delivery at any time, but this is often not the case. Our tissues are usually in a rejectivity mode, declining and forbidding toxic substances from entering. Dr. Scott explains how in this situation, cells give off parts of themselves (minerals, enzymes, and amino acids, for example) to survive and maintain status quo.

One of the main purposes of this book is to give you an understanding that what precedes sickness is an alteration in your internal environment. The body begins to lose its vitality and goes through stages of decline and decreasing resistance to toxicity, almost unnoticeably, until finally it manifests symptoms as a protective, healthy response to the disease process. With this understanding, you can use my monitoring system to balance your body's terrain, giving back your inherent power over disease. The stronger your body's response is to toxins, to pathogens' development, and to a changing terrain, the healthier you are.

This chapter approaches the cause and prevention of disease from an age-old but radically different perspective than is generally held by contemporary allopathic (that is, mainstream) medicine. Enjoy Dr. Scott's comments. He's a one-in-a-million guy who has been around for many years. He can bring the past into the future and explain the changes that healing philosophies have gone through since a few centuries back. The truth is actually the same today as it was then, and it can never be buried so deeply that we can't find it again.

The Cause and Effect of Disease: A New Perspective

When considering disease, you have to think about what's triggering the acute phenomenon you're looking at. From a nutrition-based perspective (rather than the perspective of modern allopathic medicine), the acute phenomenon is probably an indication of a hyper-sensitivity that the body has acquired as a result of a lot of defense mechanisms that have been insulted and offended.

Professor Antoine Béchamp, for example, thought that bacteria and viruses were an *effect*, not the cause, of disease. We're really a viral soup. The many viruses we're carrying around are in harmony with our bodies most of the time, living with the host organism in health. But when the manifestations of life become altered toward the direction of disease, whether by insult (such as air pollution, water pollution, food pollution, pesticides, herbicides, and the like), or by biochemical, mechanical, structural, or emotional injury, this alteration disrupts the nervous system and therefore the organism's functional capacity to adapt.

Anything that is not consistent with health becomes an influence that the organism or cell must either *adapt* to or *defend* against. (Even the adaptation mechanisms are essentially defensive in nature.) So when a practitioner of allopathic medicine looks for disease-related microorganisms in the body and then finds this organism under the microscope or isolates it by culture, he/she says, "See that? That organism is causing your disease." But that's like saying, "Those flies in the garbage can make the garbage can dirty." It's like saying that the maggots on the dead mouse killed the mouse. So it's putting the cart in front of the horse. It's confusing the whole world of biology.

In the world of biology, in the world of life, everything is fundamentally orderly. Everything is consistently predictable and reliable. So when microorganisms that are normally consistent with health and life are present, they're non-offensive. But as soon as life is altered to the extent that some element of disease is present, and the body starts defending, repairing, and healing, it produces symptoms: for instance, an abnormal secretion on its membranes. The abnormal secretion then produces, or contributes to, a change in the microorganisms. They alter their form, mutating and adapting, to be consistent with the new conditions that are present, the disease conditions. Now they're called abnormal micro-organisms, pathogens, disease-causing microbes. The typical physician says, "We have to get a drug to destroy those." And that, in allopathic medicine, is the starting point of treatment: at the disease's effect, rather than its cause. Again, this approach is like trying to kill the flies in the garbage can rather than cleaning up the garbage.

The body ultimately has to do the healing. It produces the medium, a culture for microorganisms to thrive in and propagate. When the body provides a culture in the form of abnormal (disease) secretions, then the microorganisms that propagate will be of an abnormal type, the so-called pathogens—or the garbage can example, the flies. Conventional medicine calls pathogens the cause of disease; we in holistic medicine call them the effect of disease.

The consumption of dead or dying material to support other life is a consistent principle throughout nature. Hyenas and vultures consume dead and dying animals; microorganisms consume dead and dying material. All diseased or dead life forms naturally go back to the soil, and microorganisms are the key to that process. Those microorganisms are also part of each living body, in which they consume diseased or dead forms. When death sets in, the whole body is instantaneously flooded with microorganisms—the same principle of consumption applies to the interior environment of the body and to the exterior environment of the planet. A similar principle is that when the terrain changes—internal or external—the living organisms in that environment will change.

In my early years of practice, I thought I could "remedy" people into health. The megavitamin mentality is actually very similar to the remedy mentality that pervades allopathic medicine: the belief that you can swallow something, or inject something, or cut something out, to get well. It's always a *remedy* approach rather than an *elimination of causation* approach.

It is scientific to eliminate causes. It is scientific to provide for needs. It's consistent with life to provide life's needs in accordance with its needs, not in accordance with our notions, beliefs, or superstitions. Whether you believe in megadoses of vitamins, or megadoses of drugs, or megadoses of anything, what you believe in is what you do. But if what you do doesn't work, then you'd better change your beliefs.

Today I'm not trying to dose people into health; I'm trying to nourish them into health, because nourishment is consistent with life. Many of the people I saw early in my practice actually got well much quicker when they stopped taking their vitamins and other supplements, because all these concentrated mixtures were producing intoxication and even adding to my clients' disease. Once I realized that, then all I did for thousands of people was simply to stop them from taking their vitamins and to put them on wholesome food instead. People instantly start to get better when they stop causing their own disease.

Food Is Medicine

Because we're constantly changing our internal environment with new chemicals, new poisons, and new drugs, the defense mechanisms of the body are constantly changing. Each new form of insult and assault on the living organism causes the body to go through all sorts of gyrations and defensive mechanisms to try to protect and preserve itself.

I've been in practice for forty years, and in the early years it seemed very easy to get sick people well. I used to see clients with the most horrendous diseases, "fast" them, and then "feed" them appropriately with raw fruits and vegetables, and it was miraculous to watch how these extremely ill people got well. Today, however, it's more of a struggle to get those same results.

Food has a lot to do with it. The general population's state of immunity has been offended by innumerable things from immunization and drugging to environmental insults both internal and external. As a major contributing factor to decreased immunity, I would say that the chemicalization of food has altered the responses of the human organism. We have to be more careful about the fruit we eat today, choosing organic fruit whenever possible to minimize our consumption of pesticide.

It's hard to find a pure food these days. It's also hard to find truly ripe food. Food ripened on its own tree, vine, or plant is tremendously different from food ripened after picking. That's one reason why we should be more careful in our selections of produce. Some foods are characteristically picked green and unripe; the foods characteristically picked when ripe are becoming fewer all the time.

Essentially all of life, whether we're talking about human, microbiological, animal, or plant life—any form of life—has to find its sustenance in its food. The only way to support any form of life is to maintain its nutrition. Let me distinguish between nutrition and food: food essentially provides the elements of nutrition, but nutrition supplies the needs of life. It's impossible to sustain life without good nutrition. For a period of time, you can sustain human life in a state of malnutrition, or faulty nutrition, or offended nutrition, but it's a lower quality of life, and it's usually a diseased state.

To overcome disease, we must overcome nutritional failures. One such failure is lack of excellence in the quality of available food. Another big failure is lack of excellence in the organism's digestive efficiency in translating food into usable nutrients. There's also a big failure in lack of excellence in proper excretion of the metabolic waste that is a byproduct of food-processing within the organism. So we need to deal with these areas of food, digestion, and excretion in the maintenance of healthy human life.

Food is the first line of offense in turning disease around—turning the organism around from disease to health—because there is no health problem that doesn't have an associated nutritional derangement. All of life, in all its expressions, must be maintained by the translation of food into nutrients available to every living cell in the organism.

It all comes down to intelligent selectivity and intelligent rejectivity. These are mechanisms that are preprogrammed into the organism's nutritional self-regulatory system; that is, the organism itself, even down to the cellular level, decides what foods it will accept and what it will reject. It's my observation that people who are in excellent health use a wide spectrum of foods without too much offense to the organism; but when their health breaks down or progressively deteriorates, especially in the acute phase of illness, the body rejects food totally for a period of time. For instance, during high fevers, the body doesn't want any food, as whatever is consumed at that time will only add to the fever. Then, as the organism progresses through the various stages of deterioration into degeneration and finally into terminal disease, there is a progressive failure of the organism to utilize nutrients efficiently, along with a progressive increase in the production of toxic elements from food.

Before the acute phase of illness, as the body first heads in the direction of nutritional failure, it moves in the direction of auto-intoxication or self-poisoning. The cells become weak and can't perform normal cellular functions, especially their regeneration-degeneration cycle, and toxicity builds up within and around them. The body may then selectively reject certain foods, perhaps responding to them with a hypersensitivity of some type. That is a clear signal telling you that there's a condition going on, and it's probably the earliest point at which you can start making the changes that will reverse the whole disease process. In order to restore your body's nutritional efficiency, you must address eating habits and lifestyle.

The Process of Disease

If we were to make a chart of life, with perfect health at the top of the chart and death at the bottom, rarely would an organism leap from perfect health all the way to death in an instant, except as a result of some violence or accident. But progressively, over the years, as we age and deteriorate and experience disease, we move down the chart. An initial loss of perfect health is characterized by a degree of fatigue. The cells of the organism are no longer fully restored by rest and sleep and nutrition, so now they are somewhat less efficient. We call that *enervation*. Enervation means loss of nerve energy, loss of vital energy. That's the first sign of an imbalance. As we progress downward in this chart of life toward death, we go through various stages of enervation.

The cells of the living organism progressively become more exhausted in their capability.

As vitality—the efficiency with which life carries on its processes—goes down, the exchange of nutrient utilization and excretion also goes down. Then defensive activity tends to go up, because as long as the body is alive, it will always attempt to restore balance within itself by defensive mechanisms. So it may give you a sense of fatigue, or a sense of pain, or a sense of distress in some other form. That distress is a message from the cells of your body to your brain, and now your consciousness is aware of your symptoms. But initially, it all starts with decreased vitality. You may not even be aware of that early fatigue until your vitality deteriorates further. By the time you become aware of the physical fatigue, you're probably three or four stages down the chart already.

The next stage is toxicity. When living cells become less efficient in their processes of nutrition, excretion, absorption, and utilization, plus disposal of the waste products of that metabolic process, the cells become somewhat toxic. Now they are not only enervated, they are also offended by their own waste products of nutrition, which are the byproducts of their metabolism. The consequence to a living cell of becoming toxic is that its activity becomes intensified. So it speeds up its metabolic processes to compensate for its failure, which brings the cell to a state of further excitability and irritation. This state is actually the defense mechanism of that cell responding to the toxic state.

Now comes accumulation. Months or even years have gone by and waste is starting to accumulate in the system. Next the body approaches the degenerative states. Toxemia, a condition of accumulated poisons in the body, becomes magnified. The decrease in the efficiency of the body is mirrored by an increase in intoxication from metabolic waste. Normal waste that the cells are putting out and taking in from their environment is added to the accumulation of whatever other poisons you were taking: drugs, caffeine, alcohol, pesticides, you name it. All that buildup is affecting the living cells, which respond with excitability and irritability and intoxication. If you treat these symptoms with more poisons in the form of drugs, you are only adding more defensive need to this organism.

The moment the body in high vitality is insulted and offended and toxic, it implements its defensive responses. This is not an intense attack by some outside thing called a bacterium or what have you, but rather an acute, intense defense response, which could be a high fever, a lot of vomiting, pain, an eruption on the skin, or diarrhea—some defense mechanism that says, "Get this poison out of here, and let's get back to normal and get on with life."

When you are in high vitality, your body can mobilize with tremendous intensity to deal with a toxic and offensive state immediately, but as your vitality goes down, your body becomes less efficient in its ability to mobilize its "army." The more toxic your body becomes, the more its vitality decreases, and then you are living in a lower energy state—though you may not even realize it, because it can come on so slowly. But then you move into chronic disease, which is the inability to mobilize enough defensive effort to solve the problem of increasing enervation and toxicity.

Change the Process

I'm sure that real "inherited" conditions do exist, but I think true genetic diseases or disorders are pretty rare. Unfortunately, many doctors love to tell people what they want to hear, for instance, "It's not your fault that you've got this problem, it's your grandma's fault," "It's anybody's fault but your own." But as much as some of us would like to believe it, that's not true. The only practical way you can change your organism, or change what it's doing to itself in health or disease, is to change what *you're* doing to it. Disease is a process, so *change the process.* Change what you're doing every day of your life: eating food. It's the most practical, sensible thing in this world. A lot of disease conditions can be completely avoided. You don't necessarily have to die of the same disease your parents did. You can steer clear of the causes of disease and live out a normal lifetime before the biological clock of your mortal organism finally runs down.

If you look at the processes of pathology described in the previous section, you see why we die early. More than one prominent physician has said, "It is not surprising that people die. The question is, why do they live?" The lives of many people in today's world are so pathological, so degenerative. The only way we can change that is to change the environment in which we live—mainly, our own internal environment. We can all survive quite well in an external environment that is only half-way reasonable, as long as our internal environment is properly maintained. That's where nutrition comes in; that's how to sustain life. Why destroy the clock prematurely?

A Sensitized Immune Response: The Price of Health

Once you intensify the sensitivity of your immune system, as you need to do if you want your best health, you're going to have an intensely sensitive immune response to everything that's offensive to life. That's the only way you're going to learn intellectually and intuitively how to avoid things that are offensive.

After they've been on a good diet for a long time, a lot of people say, "Jeez, I had one glass of wine/one beer/one cup of coffee/a puff off this cigarette, and my body just went crazy. I got very hyper, I got a reaction... Before, when I was using coffee/drinking beer/smoking all the time, it didn't bother me." Once you've cleaned out your system, however, the body really attacks any poisons it subsequently encounters. This reaction makes you really feel the strength and energy of your immune system's response, and that's not a bad thing—it's very important.

You have the choice of eliminating the causes of disease by building a good defensive system, or of suppressing all your symptoms with poisons called medicine. In suppressing your symptoms, however, you suppress your immune responses, and when you suppress your immune responses, you can no longer mobilize a defense effort sufficient to resolve your "poisoning."

The best way to maintain your health with an intensely sensitive immune system is by using primarily raw food in the diet. As you sustain the life principle of immunity with this nutrition, your body will then have an acute response to any toxic or offensive condition. Every time you offend, insult, or damage your organism in any way, it's going to spring instantly into defensive action, which is uncomfortable. It's going to produce symptoms. But dealing with this discomfort by taking an aspirin or some other medication is not the right approach, because that suppresses the body's defensive action and drives the offending toxins deeper into the tissues. Doing a fast, on the other hand, allows that defensive response to accomplish its purpose, which is to restore normalcy in the body.

It's so simple and logical, once you see through what you're doing to yourself. The logic is to fast a day or two, a meal or two— whatever it takes to allow the body to restore harmony again. Your organism simply wants to be happy and symptom-free during your whole lifetime, and it *can* be symptom-free unless you damage it, offend it, insult it, or do something that evokes a defensive reaction.

Symptoms are always a defense action. Symptoms are not an attack— the body doesn't attack you, your heart doesn't attack you. Your body protects you, defends you, repairs you, heals you. It always mobilizes its defense action to help you, not to destroy. Whether the symptoms are pain, swelling, fever, or anything else, there is really only one disease.

That one disease is really a defense action, and that one defense action is called inflammation. Every time a tissue is intoxicated and irritated, it will evoke the defensive action of inflammation. Inflammation is characterized by heat, redness, swelling, and pain. The pain lets the brain know there's something wrong; the fever, swelling, and redness are all parts of the immune system's response to damage. So it all goes together.

Now, if you do something to stop the inflammation, such as taking an anti-inflammatory drug, you'll be stopping the defense action, suppressing your immune system, and once again causing an accumulation of toxic waste in your cells. Then what was simply inflammation becomes an ulcer instead, because the acidity of that waste destroys the cells you were trying to heal. An example is leaky bowel syndrome, holes burned through the intestinal wall, which can result from taking anti-inflammatories. You also enter a different stage of disease—a chronic stage.

Eventually, the body tries to repair that damage by replacing the dead tissue with scars—non-functional tissues. Now you have fibrosis, or hardening of the arteries, arthritis, sclerosis of the liver or brain, or something else, from the destruction of living cells and their replacement by scar tissue. Some of the cells in the replacement tissue may mutate and form abnormal cells under these same suppressed conditions. Then some abnormal cells become tumors, and some of those tumors may become malignant, which is cancer. All as the result of interfering with the natural process of defense, repair, and healing! But instead, if you fast, and support life with nutrition, and stop offending, you allow your body to accomplish its purpose and repair the damage appropriately with its natural defense mechanisms—which, despite all of the apparent complications, is what all disease really is.

PART TWO

ProMetabolics:
Self-Monitoring and Balancing
for Optimal Health

INTRODUCTION TO THE MONITORING SYSTEM AND BALANCING YOUR pH

Now that you've read Part One, you have a new understanding of how disease develops. Whether you're ill or well, it is always important to know what's going on inside your body. The way to reverse the process of disease is to restore the balance of your internal terrain. Here in Part Two, I describe a self-monitoring system using pH, body temperature, and blood pressure readings to do just that.

Monitoring and balancing your pH as detailed in this chapter builds your health from the cells up. Cells make up tissues, which make up organs, which make up systems, so your whole body responds. The next chapter describes how to monitor your temperature and blood pressure, so you can observe and address the functioning of your hormonal system—a very important component of your terrain. Using this system is fun and easy, and it puts you in control of your body and health.

An Individualized Approach to Your Health

Because you are a one-of-a-kind snowflake, your health is an individual proposition. The ProMetabolics monitoring system is a unique approach to health. A main advantage of this system is that you are freed from the limitations of any one-size-fits-all program. And as your terrain is always changing—especially during disease—whatever diet or supplements you choose can be monitored and modified accordingly. This system will help you know your body better than any physician does.

What are the benefits of using this system?

- If you are healthy, it helps you stay healthy.
- If you are undergoing detoxification, it helps you watch the process so you don't become too acidic or develop nutrient deficiencies.

- It helps you identify any special supplements you may need and helps you determine the proper dosages.
- If you are sick, whether with a cold, sub-clinical symptoms, or chronic illness, it supports and speeds your recovery.
- It helps you assess your metabolism's response to foods so you can determine what foods are good for you and what foods to avoid.
- It helps your body recover from work-outs or injury.
- If you are interested in losing excess weight, it helps you balance gland activity and choose the right foods for healthy weight loss.
- It helps you regulate your hormones. This is especially beneficial for athletes, as well as for menopause in women and andropause in men.

This system does not lie or mislead you, and it gives you feedback during the early stages of any nutritional approach, so you can head off a problem before it happens. Taking a particular supplement for a given condition or following a particular diet could be either right or wrong for you. You could, for example, be taking ginseng to elevate your mood and energy; however, it could also be raising your blood pressure and overworking your adrenal glands—and the monitoring system will tell you. You could be an athlete eating extra protein while you're training; however, too much protein could be creating an unhealthy acidic condition—and the monitoring system will tell you.

You won't be using this system to diagnose and treat a specific disease as in conventional medicine. You'll be observing and monitoring your body's own processes, with the goal of keeping your terrain in balance so your systems can function normally. You'll be giving your body the nutrients it needs and watching as it heals itself. One client of mine, for example, simply took iodine to support her thyroid because of her low temperature, and her panic attacks, allergies, and migraines disappeared as well. Just balance and observe.

I have seen this system in action for twenty-five years and it works! It's in line with the Chinese philosophy that disease is really nothing but an imbalance in the body's nutrients and energy. Giving every manifestation of imbalance a disease name such as fibromyalgia, arthritis, and cancer can be scary and defeating; a name also gives false specificity, as if only one part of the body is involved, as if heart disease is only in the heart. In reality, every illness, right down to the common cold, involves the whole body and every part of its metabolism. It takes months, even years to get sick, and never is only one part of the body ill. This is why I am encouraging you to think in terms of wholism, of the interconnections and interdependence throughout your body.

Introduction to Your pH

All substances in nature have a pH. The abbreviation stands for "potential of hydrogen," which can be translated as the concentration of hydrogen ions in whatever solution or other sample is being considered (for example, blood, urine, saliva, coffee, or soda). It is measured on a scale from zero to 14.0; in general terms, on that scale, 7 is neutral, a pH above 7 is alkaline, and a pH below 7 is acidic. Acidosis is a state of greater-than-normal acidity in the body's fluids and/or tissues, and alkalosis is a state of greater-than-normal alkalinity. Neither state is optimal for health.

The metabolic and enzymatic reactions in your body occur at various pH levels. Your stomach, for instance, sets up an acidic pH environment for protein digestion; however, your small intestine is alkaline, as are your pancreatic secretions and your gall bladder's bile. If any of those required pHs are affected by poor diet, practically any digestive or intestinal illness can manifest. Similarly, your circulating blood's normal pH range is 7.35–7.45, and if the blood's pH deviates by only a bit, say down to 6.95, this can lead to something as drastic as a coma. Clearly, your body needs to regulate its pH in order to function properly and maintain health.

As you might imagine, your diet has an enormous effect on your pH. Unfortunately, our society promotes the widespread and frequent consumption of acid-producing foods and beverages. On top of that, add some of the other things that acidify the body—stress, environmental toxins, medications, even exercise—and you're likely to wind up in an acidic state, which has many negative effects on the body and can lead to serious health problems.

People are seldom found to be overly alkaline, but it can happen. If you're on a vegetarian or vegan diet, you may become too alkaline, and that's not good either, as it can lead to a protein deficiency and other problems. In my practice, I see alkaline pH in vegetarians who are protein-deficient, unhealthy, and weak—I was one of these people once, and I looked like a chicken without feathers.

Your internal terrain is primarily fluids such as blood, secretions (throughout the digestive tract and from the pancreas), and lymph fluid. All of your cells, glands, enzymes, and systems function at their best when the pH of that terrain is normal. Your salivary and urinary pH reflect whether your terrain is balanced, how good your diet is, whether you're digesting your foods properly, how your body is responding to nutritional supplements, and more—so an increase or decrease in your pH readings provides very important information.

Minerals: Your pH-Buffering System

Humans have a few built-in mechanisms for eliminating excess acids from the body. Your kidneys' main function is to filter the bloodstream, and they have "the final say" in excreting acidic and alkaline substances as needed to balance the blood's pH. Your lungs assist by eliminating carbonic acid into the air as you exhale—that's why exercise and yoga breathing exercises can also help balance your blood's pH.

But the main mechanism of your pH-regulating system is found both inside and outside of your cells, in the form of alkaline minerals. Buffers are substances that help balance the pH of a solution by counteracting acidity. Alkaline minerals including sodium, potassium, calcium, and magnesium act as buffers in your terrain to keep your blood and tissues at their appropriate pH. Much of the body's mineral reserves are stored within the bones. As your tissues and blood become acidic, minerals are released from storage to neutralize the acids and also to help kick them out through the liver and kidneys.

If you run low on minerals because of a poor diet, acids accumulate in your body, get deposited into various tissues, and cause pain and inflammation. Acidosis also promotes the development of your body's normal microbial population into bacterial, viral, and fungal infections. To reverse these processes, you need to take in more minerals. But just as your stored minerals affect your terrain's pH, your pH also affects your ability to obtain minerals from diet and supplements. That's because minerals are best assimilated by the body under specific pH conditions.

For example, iodine is assimilated in a narrow pH range of 6.3–6.6. (If you're not absorbing enough iodine from your food for your thyroid to function properly, would you want to take a drug that can acidify your terrain, or would you rather balance your pH for optimum iodine absorption?) Selenium is best absorbed in a pH range of 6.2–6.9; zinc and copper, 6.1–6.8; and potassium and calcium, 5.8–7.2 (this is also the same range for most of the B-vitamins). Magnesium and silica are absorbed in a wider pH range, 5.6–7.4.

The body's minerals are constantly being released into the blood to neutralize the acid wastes that your cells are constantly producing. With increased acidification due to diet, age, stress, or over-exercise, your buffering system is overtaxed. The resulting depletion of your calcium, magnesium, potassium, and sodium reserves can lead to fatigue, slow recovery, muscle cramps, injury, osteoporosis...the list goes on. (It is one of the major reasons why elderly people have such brittle bones.)

Furthermore, when the terrain is acidic and acids aren't being eliminated in a timely fashion, toxins are stored around cells called the mesenchyme, in muscles and joints. As time goes on, toxins get deeper into the cells and even displace your stored minerals.

Diet, pH, and Digestion

The typical American diet is full of acid-producing foods and beverages. If you eat a highly acidic and acid-forming meal—hot dogs, soda, and French fries, for instance—your mineral buffer system must immediately go to work to neutralize the acids. (Most fruits and vegetables, by contrast, are alkalizing to the body.) This type of diet is one of the major reasons why people become so mineral-deficient over time. Plus, because we don't eat enough raw foods, which would provide us with additional digestive enzymes, our body's own supply of digestive enzymes is drained and depleted, making our digestion inefficient and incomplete. These factors produce an overly acidic state.

To digest certain proteins such as the gluten in wheat and the casein in milk, the stomach must secrete large amounts of hydrochloric acid (HCl). That requires the pancreas to release even more of the secretions that are needed to alkalize these stomach acids farther down the digestive tract. This burden lays the foundation for all sorts of pancreatic problems to set in when the organ's natural functioning is disturbed by a poor diet over a long period. Different people experience different symptoms: pancreatic insufficiency, pancreatitis, and pancreatic enzyme deficiencies, for example. Taking antacids doesn't correct the problem. But if the diet is corrected, these conditions may be reversed. (When my dog was diagnosed with pancreatic insufficiency, my veterinarian had the insight to prescribe digestive enzymes. I wonder what your doctor would give you for a pancreatic problem...)

Becoming Acidic: A Downward Spiral

Acidification often starts from taking in too many acid-forming foods and beverages: excessive protein, dairy products, alcohol, coffee, cooked grains and refined flour, sugar and other sweeteners, beer, wine, chocolate... The body's overload of acid wastes is dumped into the bloodstream to be eliminated through the kidneys, bowels, lungs, skin, and any open orifice. These organs and orifices can get overworked or congested with toxins, drugs, and mucus, and symptoms begin to manifest. Early stages of this pH imbalance present themselves as a cold, a flu, and/or sinus congestion.

If you get into a continually acidic state, your kidneys become overburdened with acid wastes. Eventually, their filtering mechanisms begin to wear out. (Weakened kidneys are one of the biomarkers or biological signposts of aging; fortunately, kidney failure is an aging process over which you have some control.) When the kidneys are overloaded, toxins remain in the bloodstream and travel around the body, affecting the normally alkaline environment of your cells and initiating the deterioration of organs and tissues. You can see how important it is to supply the minerals utilized by your buffering system. When you consider the state of our mineral-deficient soil and food as well as nutrient loss from cooking, you begin to wonder how we live as long as we do.

The blood then pulls minerals out of the body's tissues to neutralize the acids. Because these minerals are taken away from their ordinary functions, deficiencies arise in other areas. When the tissues become deficient in minerals, the body robs calcium from the bones as an extra buffer. This is something you don't want to occur, because as previously noted, this scenario is behind arthritic pain, inflammatory disease, and osteoporosis. At this point, the body is in need of more potassium and magnesium and other minerals to stop this degenerative process.

As minerals become depleted, acids circulating in the bloodstream are redeposited into the tissues, beginning an inflammatory process in the joints. Other symptoms such as swelling, inflammation, aches and pains, fibromyalgia, eczema, acne, boils, cramps, and headaches develop. As the overload of acids gets worse, they're stored in tissues and organs throughout your body and even your brain. Many of these acids (and other toxins) are stored in your fatty tissues; this has a lot to do with weight gain, because the body creates more fat cells to harbor the toxins and also holds on to excess water to dilute their acidity.

Stress on the pH buffering system also affects respiration—even down to the cellular level. Inhalation brings oxygen, which is alkaline, into the bloodstream, and exhalation releases carbon dioxide and carbonic acid into the air. When the body becomes acidic, the excess hydrogen ions prompt the brain's respiratory controls to increase the respiration rate for faster discharge of carbon dioxide to help restore terrain pH. (If the body becomes alkaline, the respiration rate decreases to retain more carbon dioxide.) So if your blood and lungs are working to buffer and eliminate excess acids, but you're smoking at the same time, that's a big mistake—not only are you undermining your body's efforts by smoking, you're possibly setting the stage for lung disease.

Oxygen is absorbed within the pH range of 5.3–7.6. As your terrain becomes more acidic, your cells get less oxygen. Going down any further than 5.3 results in fermentation and even less oxygen absorption. Cells respirate, "breathe in and breathe out," in their own fashion. They expand in the oxidation phase, which is when their fuel combines with oxygen and is burned to power their activities; then they contract in the reduction phase and return to normal before respirating again. Each cell in your body must carry out three basic functions: repair, replace, and eliminate/detoxify. If any of these functions are inhibited, the cell malfunctions, and its relationships with other cells are also affected. If there's not enough oxygen in the blood to support cellular respiration, all cell functions begin to change and compensate for that deficit.

The body always tries to maintain a yin-yang balance. So when a molecule of acid is deposited into the tissues, the body compensates by releasing an alkaline molecule back into the bloodstream. As the tissues are overloaded with acids, the tissue pH decreases; and as the blood responds by taking minerals from tissues and bones, the blood pH increases, becoming more alkaline. Minerals that were drawn from the tissues leave the body through the urine, but sodium is retained in the blood to help escort acid wastes coming from the tissues.

When the blood becomes more alkaline from its increased mineral content, the red blood cells begin to absorb more oxygen. You'd think this would be a good thing, wouldn't you? However, an overload of acids in the tissues and a dumping of alkaline minerals into the blood create what is called the Buhr effect: with rising blood alkalinity, the red blood cells get saturated with too much oxygen but then can't release it back to the tissues. It's complicated to explain, but in a nutshell, when the pH is off-kilter, certain biochemical exchanges in the body don't happen the way they should. The result of the red blood cells' inability to release oxygen is a low-oxygen or anaerobic environment in the tissues.

Remember what you learned in Part One about an acidic, low-oxygen internal environment? Now the pleomorphic party begins…

Acidity, Microorganisms, and Disease

As you read in Part One, proto-microbes called endobiants normally live symbiotically with your cells and have the ability to change their form relative to the terrain. They have been observed, when subjected to a drastic pH change, to pass through several stages and become pathogenic or "disease-causing" organisms—bacterial, viral, and fungal forms—to survive. As your terrain acidifies, your body's endobiants begin to cycle upward into their pathogenic forms: yeast, bacteria, and fungus.

During the acidification process, the blood's oxygen level is lowering, so the body's cells are becoming oxygen-deprived, and basic cellular functions are being hindered. As Nobel Laureate Dr. Otto Warburg stated, "When the pH is off and our bodies are becoming more acidic, our cells get less oxygen. Cancer thrives under an acid tissue pH/oxygen-deficient environment." (*Warburg O. The Metabolism of Tumours. Arnold Constable Press, London, UK, 1930.*) Is it any wonder that cancer rates today are so high?

In this acidic, low-oxygen environment, the endobiant begins to evolve up its life cycle to save itself. Instead of remaining a "normal" organism that uses oxygen to burn fuel aerobically, it becomes an anaerobic, fermenting organism that doesn't need oxygen—it becomes yeast, or another kind of fungus, or mold. Given that cancer cells thrive in an anaerobic environment, what do you think a cancer cell is? It's essentially a fermenting entity, much like a fungus. (The endobiant fungus form is called mucor racemusus fresen. If you take cells from a cancer tumor and culture them, guess what you find in the culture? The fungus mucor racemusus fresen.)

Although the medical establishment says there are hundreds of strains of virus and bacteria, those are not actually separate entities; they are simply the different cycles of growth that endobiants go through. Killing a given kind of microbe at any one stage of its existence isn't going to kill all of them, only the microbes at that particular stage. Those at a different point in their life cycle continue to grow, scavenging the protein wastes from damaged cells for nourishment. It sounds to me as though such an approach only makes things worse.

As I've said, you normally live in symbiosis with your microbes. But at this point, the overgrowth of yeast and fungus in your body is feeding on protein and sugar and poisoning the terrain with secreted wastes called mycotoxins. Mycotoxins are one of the main causes of allergies and chemical sensitivities. The body becomes overburdened with acids from these microbial wastes, which stress your immune system and can overstimulate your thyroid and adrenals. The exhaustion of these systems results in more weight gain, more allergies, and more chemical sensitivities.

Some mycotoxins also break down nerve tissue and interfere with nerve transmission, particularly in the brain. The mycotoxin acetaldehyde, for example, is created by yeast's fermentation of alcohol and/or sugar, as happens in a severe case of Candida. An acetaldehyde overload results in anxiety, paranoia, weakness, fatigue, loss of mental concentration, and total lack of ambition—this "spaced-out" feeling is not pleasant, believe me. Meanwhile, acidification continues, and your systems are in disarray because the terrain's pH has been thrown off. By now, you may be experiencing symptoms such as vaginal itch, mucus discharge, rectal itching, prostatitis, ringworm, premenstrual syndrome, fungus under the nails, moles, skin spots, impotence, and more.

Every symptom imaginable can result from the causal chain that began with acidity: 1) pH changes, 2) pleomorphism leading to the fungus form, 3) immune system overload, and 4) adrenal and thyroid overstimulation and exhaustion. An entire cascade of symptoms is produced by a toxic cycle of acidic wastes: your cells excrete citric and lactic acid wastes, your diet brings in more acid, and your microbes then produce their own acids. The particular symptoms that result are in accordance with your genetic make-up and how much accumulated waste your body can handle.

According to the scientist Günther Enderlein, all chronic diseases are based on endobiants' development into higher forms that have a pathogenic relationship with their host, as they develop their own metabolism that poisons the host's body fluids, primarily by lactic acid production: "Basically, there is not a multitude of diseases, but only one constitutional disease, namely the constant over-acidification of the blood, which disturbs the central regulation of the body, disorienting it, all of which is mainly the result of an inverted way of living and eating."

In 1924 Dr. Warburg clearly demonstrated that cancerous tumors contain up to ten times the amount of lactic acid found in healthy human tissues. This created acidity reacts chemically with iron, causing the blood's hemoglobin (which utilizes iron) to lose some of its ability to collect oxygen from the lungs. The result is a lower oxygen level in the bloodstream, so less oxygen is available to the cells in the body's tissues. Reduced oxygen sets the stage for cells to replace their normal aerobic means of energy production, which involves oxygen and the "tiny furnaces" called mitochondria, by turning to fermentation instead. The ongoing acidity and fermentation lead to protein deficiencies and free radical activity—and stimulate endobiants to become pathogenic.

pH, Minerals, and Your Nervous System

When your pH is out of balance or your buffering minerals are depleted, your body and health are affected in many ways—even your nervous system and emotional balance are affected. As you may already know, the nervous system has two main parts: the cerebrospinal division and the autonomic division. This book is chiefly concerned with the autonomic division, which is not only the master regulator of metabolism but also controls all the involuntary activities of the body: heart beat, respiration, digestion, tissue growth and repair, temperature, hormone secretion, and many, many more functions.

The autonomic division also has two parts: the sympathetic and parasympathetic systems. They are dualistic opposites and counterbalance each other—yin-yang, if you will—just as everything in the universe needs its counterbalance to achieve balance. The sympathetic system "turns on" the energy-utilizing organs and glands such as the adrenals, thyroid, and pituitary; it prepares your body for "fight-or-flight." The parasympathetic nervous system turns on the organs and glands pertaining to digestion, elimination, repair, and rebuilding; it's responsible for energy-conserving processes and causes you to rest.

The table below gives examples of how the two parts work together in a synchronized fashion to regulate various involuntary processes.

Sympathetic-Controlled	Parasympathetic-Controlled
Pupils dilate	Pupils contract
Heart rate increases	Heart rate decreases
Intestinal functions slow down	Intestinal functions speed up
Bladder contracts	Bladder relaxes
Liver releases glucose	Liver stores glucose
Stomach decreases digestive secretions	Stomach increases digestive secretions

Not surprisingly, both the sympathetic and parasympathetic systems are influenced by the body's mineral status, as there are specific minerals that stimulate and balance each one. This is where your pH and your nervous system intersect, because some of those minerals are the same ones that make up your pH buffering system:

- Sodium – the principle ion in the fluid outside of the body's cells, essential to nerve transmission and muscle contraction
- Potassium – the principle mineral inside the body's cells, helps maintain nerve transmission and muscle contraction; potassium and sodium briefly trade places across cell membranes to control muscle contraction and maintain a steady heart beat

- Calcium – participates in muscle contraction as well as blood clotting and nerve transmission
- Magnesium – participates in hundreds of enzyme reactions, necessary for cellular energy production; with calcium, involved in muscle contraction, blood clotting, and a dynamic interaction that helps regulate blood pressure and lung function

Three of those major minerals play roles of paramount importance to your autonomic activity: sodium stimulates the sympathetic system; potassium stimulates the parasympathetic system; and calcium regulates or balances both systems. So you can see that both systems need minerals to help maintain their proper balance, and a deficiency in the proper minerals will create an imbalance between the two. The table below shows some of the symptoms that can result from such an imbalance.

Sympathetic-Dominant Symptoms	Parasympathetic-Dominant Symptoms
Indigestion	Loose bowels
High blood pressure	Low blood sugar
Insomnia	Irregular heart beat
High motivation level	Chronic fatigue
Irritability	Lethargy
Good concentration	Procrastination

Let's say your diet contains a lot of sodium, possibly creating a state of sympathetic dominance. As you've heard, sodium can cause high blood pressure; it contracts the blood vessels and is also dehydrating, so your body cramps and gets thirsty, and your blood pressure goes up. People with high blood pressure and high-sodium diets are often angry, irritated, and uptight. Their adrenals are always kicked into high gear, and they are "fast burners" in terms of metabolism. To restore balance, you would need to reduce your sodium intake, drink more water, and adjust your diet until the monitoring system shows that your readings have normalized.

As another example, let's say your blood pressure is too low, indicating a possible state of parasympathetic dominance. You can try increasing your intake of sodium-rich foods and Celtic Sea Salt® (described later in this chapter) and decreasing your intake of potassium-rich foods. If this doesn't work, you may be deficient in several minerals, and I would suggest using a multimineral supplement with sea vegetables (such as algae and seaweed) and/or a green food concentrate. (Seaweed and green foods are discussed later; see also the Juice Plus+® chapter.) Having low blood pressure, though, doesn't necessarily mean that you're high in potassium. The monitoring system will help by indicating what major minerals may be deficient and how to balance your mineral needs.

Getting Started with pH Monitoring

It's necessary to learn how to use the whole monitoring system if you want to analyze your whole-body processes, but before putting the entire puzzle together, it's easier to learn how to take each reading one by one, beginning with pH.

For your first monitoring period, you're going to take your pH readings three times per day for three to five consecutive days—five days are better, but three will do. You'll need some pH paper, which is hard to find, so here are two sources I recommend: Bert's Pharmacy (570-888-2157) and Micro Essential Lab (718-338-3618).

Whole foods and whole-food concentrates such as Juice Plus+® are what I call "foundational nutrition" (described later in the book). If you have been taking Juice Plus+®, it doesn't interfere with the monitoring system to keep taking it prior to and during a monitoring period; but don't start taking it, or any new supplement, two days before monitoring or during monitoring. It is important, however, to stop taking all non-foundational supplements (that is, amino acids, minerals, vitamins, glandular formulas, and the like) for two full days and nights before you begin monitoring. Your terrain and metabolism will then be "at norm" in their unaffected states, so you can assess them clearly and respond appropriately if needed—the system will show you what to do.

How to Measure Your pH

As you might imagine, your saliva is closely related to your blood and your digestive system. The pH of your saliva is an indicator of how your liver, stomach, and other digestive organs are reacting to diet or stress, as well as to supplements or medications or illness. The pH of your urine also indicates how your body is processing food and supplements.

Testing your pH is quite simple. After you do it once or twice as follows, you'll get it:

- To test your saliva, put a small piece of pH paper in your mouth, wet it well with your saliva, and wait ten seconds. Then remove it, and match it to one of the colors on the pH paper's container; these colors correspond to pH values, also shown on the container. Write down your saliva's pH value.
- To test your urine, dip another piece of pH paper directly into your urine stream as you urinate. Do not use a cup or other container, as it could affect your reading. Wait ten seconds, match the color on the pH paper to a color on the container as before, and write down your urine's pH value.

Normal pH. Normal pH readings for both saliva and urine are in the range of 6.5–6.8. Readings deviate relative to your health status and the foods and supplements you're taking into your body. Both salivary and urinary pH values also vary somewhat depending on the time of day. Your morning readings, for example, will differ a bit from your readings later on, as morning pH reflects how the body has handled the night's fasting and cleansing cycle. (This is discussed further in the next section.)

Timing matters. You should take your salivary and urinary pH readings at the same time. Suggested testing times are 8:00 a.m., 2:00 p.m., and 8:00 p.m., but you can tailor these times to your own daily schedule, according to the following guidelines:

- Take your morning reading as soon as you wake up. (If you're curious, you can take another reading two hours after breakfast to see which way the meal pushed your pH.)
- For your midday and evening readings, it's best to wait at least two hours after any meal or snack before testing your pH; the readings will then tell you how you're processing that meal.
- At night, don't eat anything within three hours before bedtime, or your next morning's pH won't reflect the night's detoxification results—instead, it will reflect your body's response to its last meal or snack. Your body conducts its natural cleansing functions at night while you sleep, and you don't want to interfere with that cycle or to produce and retain excess acid wastes overnight. In the evening, drink plenty of water and minimize your intake of fruit juice (and fruit). (I like to eat dinner at 5:00 or 6:00 p.m. and then have only water or fresh vegetable juice after that; mixed cucumber, celery, and a small amount of apple juice is a nice alkaline drink in the evening.)

If your pH changes like a teeter-totter according to your meals and other factors, don't be alarmed. Averaging your readings over a few days gives you a clearer picture of your terrain (an averaging method is shown later). If either of your pH indicators remains too acidic or too alkaline for too long, then you need to do something about it. But don't worry—figuring out how to balance your pH is not difficult. The ProMetabolics Terrain-Balancing Chart in this chapter will tell you what to do.

Monitoring Your Health: pH over the Course of the Day

For the most part, what you are observing in the variations of your urinary and salivary pH throughout the day is the effect that foods and other substances have on your body. Specifically, you can see whether they've produced an acidifying or alkalinizing reaction that has caused your terrain to be too acidic or too alkaline relative to its optimum pH range of 6.5–6.8. Stress and other emotional states can also affect the body's pH; for instance, a nervous, uptight person typically burns sugar rapidly and can create an acidic condition by doing so.

This section describes normal morning, midday, and evening pH readings, and what it may mean if your readings deviate from those norms. Please note, however, that one day's pH readings aren't enough information for general monitoring; you really need at least three days' worth of this "data" to see a full, accurate picture of your terrain's pH and, if it shows an imbalance, to choose the appropriate course of action for adjusting it.

Morning pH. Although you may find your morning pH readings to be the same for both saliva and urine, it's usually normal for morning saliva to be slightly alkaline and morning urine to be slightly acidic relative to the ideal pH range of 6.5–6.8. A salivary pH of 7.0 is a little high but still acceptable for the morning. A somewhat acidic urinary pH in the morning, at 6.5 or a little lower, simply reflects that the body is excreting a whole night's worth of waste products and indicates that the kidneys are keeping up with the liver in eliminating these wastes.

If your morning urine is above 6.5, and especially if it's approaching 7.0, this is a classic sign that acids are building up in the liver or elsewhere rather than being excreted through the urine.

Midday pH. Midday saliva readings should be in the normal range of 6.5–6.8, showing that your body has finished cleaning out the night's waste. By midday, your urinary pH should also come up to the normal range (best at 6.5) and then be in that range during the rest of the day.

If your midday urinary pH has not risen from the morning's acidity into the normal range, it means you ate acid-producing foods for breakfast, or your body has not yet expelled all of its acid wastes from the day before.

If your midday urinary pH is alkaline, you may be eating too many alkaline foods and minerals and not digesting protein.

Evening pH. Evening salivary and urinary pH may be in the normal 6.5–6.8 range, rise toward the neutral point of 7.0, or become slightly more acidic, which indicates that the body is beginning its nighttime cleansing and detoxification cycle.

If your salivary pH remains acidic through the day and into the evening for three days, this means your diet is too acid-forming or your liver is retaining acid wastes, and your digestive system needs help.

If your midday and evening saliva are less alkaline than your midday and evening urine for three days, be suspicious. This relationship indicates that you're not eliminating wastes properly and are retaining acids and extra fluid.

A note on mixed acidic and alkaline pH readings. If your daily average salivary pH is acidic and your daily average urinary pH is alkaline for more than three days in a row, this is a sign that you are retaining acid, particularly in your liver and bloodstream. If you have alkaline saliva and acidic urine, you're not digesting protein properly.

How Often to Monitor—in Sickness, in Health, and in Athletes

Please don't worry that this is going to be a lot of work, because it really isn't. When you're healthy, you only need a three- to five-day monitoring period every one or two months. But you can use the monitoring system whenever you want to; for example, to make sure that your dietary and supplementation program is not throwing you out of balance.

If you're chronically ill, you'll want to monitor your pH more often. And during colds, flu, fever, or other acute illnesses, you should take your pH readings three times a day on each day that you're experiencing any symptoms. Regular, frequent monitoring during illness is important so you can make the appropriate pH-balancing adjustments to support your recovery. When you're sick, your body needs to rest, so I recommend giving your digestive system a break by fasting for one or two days on only water, fruit, and vegetable juices.

You can also check your pH readings whenever you'd like to see how a particular food, supplement, medication, or event has influenced your biochemistry. Experiment by eating and testing one food at a time, or eat and test a meal, for example, that's all protein foods or all fruits. Simply take your readings before you eat the food of interest, wait two hours, and then take your readings again to see its effect on your pH. You can do the same with supplements by first discontinuing whatever you're taking for three days, adding one supplement at a time back into your regime, taking it for two days, and then testing your pH. The food or supplement isn't good for you if it makes one or both of your pH readings too acidic or too alkaline (or if it negatively affects your body temperature or blood pressure; see the next chapter). It is good for you—or at least not bad for you—if it balances you, or alters your readings only slightly or not at all.

Although exercising is one of the greatest things you can do for your health, like everything else it has an opposite effect if not kept in balance. Training can age you rapidly if you don't attend to your body's signals. When you train, your muscles produce lactic acid. High-protein foods and drinks also create acid. In the long run, you become alkaline and mineral-deficient, and your muscles and joints always seem to be sore.

If you're an active athlete consuming lots of protein and taking amino acids (or taking steroids, which I am NOT suggesting to do!), you should take your pH readings more often: for example, two days in a row every two weeks. At times, you'll have to beef up on minerals or lay off protein—your monitoring will tell you what you need. If you get into a highly acidic state but don't want to give up protein because you want to make the front cover of a muscle magazine, you're asking for trouble. I'd rather look good and stay pain-free my whole life than look good while I'm young but live in pain when I'm older. Don't let bad advice and your ego get in the way of common sense. Let your body be your guide.

Calculating Your pH Averages

There may be certain days when you want to observe the pH effects of a particular food or supplement or to adjust your pH while you're sick. But in general, you'll drive yourself crazy if you try to monitor and balance your pH on a daily basis.

The simplest way to evaluate your pH is to average your readings over a set monitoring period. The example below illustrates an easy averaging method for a three-day monitoring period:

1. For each monitoring period day, calculate your day's average:

Time	Salivary pH reading
8:00 a.m.	6.3
2:00 p.m.	6.0
8:00 p.m.	5.5

Total these values: 6.3 + 6.0 + 5.5 = 17.8
Divide the total by the number of readings: 17.8 / 3 = 5.93
Your salivary pH average on this day is 5.9.

2. At the end of the monitoring period, average your averages:

Day	Salivary pH average
Mon.	5.9
Tues.	6.0
Wed.	7.0

Total these values: 5.9 + 6.0 + 7.0 = 18.9
Divide the total by the number of days: 18.9 / 3 = 6.3
Your three-day salivary pH average is 6.3.

Apply this averaging method separately to your salivary readings and your urinary readings. Your calculated averages reflect your pH pattern for the observation period.

As you now know, many factors can produce an acidic or alkaline pH. You don't want to remain in an overly acidic or overly alkaline state for any longer than three to five days if you can help it. If either of your calculated averages indicates a pH imbalance, consult the ProMetabolics Terrain-Balancing Chart below.

ProMetabolics Terrain-Balancing Chart

	Detox	Amino Acids	Sodium	Potassium	Adrenal Support	Iodine	HCl	Enzymes	Celtic Sea Salt®	Seaweed	Green Foods + Juices	Minerals
1. Saliva – Acidic / Urine – Alkaline	X (Liver)							X			X	
2. Saliva – Alkaline / Urine – Acidic		X					X	X	X			
3. Saliva – Acidic / Urine – Acidic	X							X			X	X
4. Saliva – Alkaline / Urine – Alkaline		X					X	X	X			
5. Saliva – Acidic / Urine – Normal	X (Liver)							X	X		X	X
6. Saliva – Normal / Urine – Acidic	X (Kidney)							X	X		X	X
Temperature – High		X				X		X	X		X	
Temperature – Low		X				X		X	X	X	X	
Blood Pressure – High			Decrease	Increase				X			X	
Blood Pressure – Low		X	Increase		X			X	X		X	

Consulting the ProMetabolics Terrain-Balancing Chart

Down the left side of the chart are the personal characteristics that you'll be monitoring: salivary and urinary pH, body temperature, and blood pressure. If any of these indicators show an imbalance, you should first try to balance your terrain by using foods. Specific supplements, shown across the top of the chart, can also be taken when necessary. You can find descriptions of the appropriate foods and suggested supplements in this chapter and also in Part Four of this book.

As an example, let's say your salivary three-day average pH is 6.1, which is acidic, and your urinary three-day average pH is 6.8, which is in the normal range. Find the box in the left-hand column of the chart that corresponds to your averages: category 5, which says "Saliva – Acidic" and "Urine – Normal." Now, going to the right along that row, the Xs indicate what you can use to balance your pH; in this case, detoxification, digestive enzymes, green foods and juices, and minerals are suggested.

If you try to balance your pH through your diet and supplements but find that you can't, this means your endocrine system is involved in the imbalance: specifically, your adrenals, thyroid, and/or pituitary. You'll want to take a deeper look into your terrain by monitoring your temperature and blood pressure (discussed in the next chapter). A pH reading can be persistently acidic, for example, if you have high blood pressure indicating imbalanced adrenal activity. You can use the monitoring system to help track down the problem, or you can simply use it to balance your whole-body metabolic processes and watch your body heal itself—this is what I mean by ProMetabolics.

If you try to balance your pH with the monitoring system for a prolonged period and you're still having trouble with it, this might indicate a chronic condition of some kind, and you should consider seeing a healthcare practitioner.

Using Food to Balance Your pH

Yin and yang, hot and cold, acid and alkaline—these opposites balance each other. The principle of eating acidifying or alkalizing foods to modify your pH is simple. If you check the pH of your urine and saliva and find them both to be acidic, you know not to eat more acid-producing foods; instead, it would be best to eat alkaline foods to restore your proper pH. (The main reason why people often get tired after meals is that instead of eating what their bodies need, they inadvertently eat the opposite.)

Below are lists of acidifying and alkalizing foods to help you balance your terrain's pH through your diet. (For additional food lists, check out *The Acid-Alkaline Food Guide* by Susan Brown and Larry Trivieri, from Square One Publishers, or see www.trans4mind.com/nutrition/pH.html.)

Acidifying Foods

All grains (except millet)
All meat and poultry
Seafood
Dairy foods (milk, butter, cream, cheese)
Eggs
Most nuts

Most oils
Animal fats
Dried peas
Dried beans
Lentils
Hulled sesame seeds

Alkalizing Foods

Most vegetables
Most fruits (fresh or dried)
Sprouts from most legumes
Soybean sprouts
Sunflower sprouts
All grasses (wheat grass, spirulina, barley)
Dandelion
Millet
Almonds
Peaches

Endive
Romaine
Tomatoes
Celery
Cucumbers
Carrots
Onions
Avocadoes
Olive oil
Unhulled sesame seeds

A note about eating fruit. Fruit usually (though not always) has an alkalizing effect and also helps with detoxification. Citrus fruits, however, are not the best choice when your urinary pH is lower than 6.5; although they are alkalizing, they have acids in them as well. Experiment with various fruits by taking your readings two hours after eating them (one at a time) to find out what works for you.

If your morning urine is overly acidic for a few days, try eating fruit for breakfast. If you have been acidic for a long time, though, you may not properly metabolize the acids and sugars in fruits, which can then make you more acidic. Sometimes with difficult acidic conditions it's best to have vegetables—maybe steamed vegetables, vegetable broth, or a green drink—for breakfast instead of fruit:.

Because fruits are often grown in mineral-deficient soils or shipped unripe from remote places, it's best to eat fruits that are organically grown and indigenous to your climate region, so they are as nutrient-rich as they ought to be and ripened naturally instead of artificially while in transit.

pH and Detoxification

The ProMetabolics Terrain-Balancing Chart suggests detoxification for several of the six pH categories, including the three with an acidic salivary pH (categories 1, 3, and 5). Acidic saliva indicates that the liver is holding on to acids and the digestive system is not breaking foods down properly.

In general, detoxification is primarily for the liver, but it can also cleanse the bloodstream and all other organs. Many detox methods exist and many herbal detox formulas are available. Finding what works best for you requires experimentation, but it is well worthwhile. (See the Environmental and Heavy Metal Toxicity chapter for information on far-infrared saunas, Metal-Free®, and other detox methods.)

People are often mineral-deficient before starting a detox program. During detoxification, buffering minerals from the body's reserves are used to neutralize toxins as they are released from the tissues and flushed out, so you may need to rebalance your pH afterward. Surprisingly, sometimes it is necessary to eat more protein during detox, because protein provides sulfur-containing amino acids that are needed to open up detoxification pathways in the body.

When you're detoxifying, your urine may briefly be acidified by the toxins exiting your body. In such a case, you can use concentrated alfalfa, the algae chlorella or spirulina, carrot juice, or other alkaline foods to balance your body chemistry. Two excellent formulas to support detox are Liver Liquid and Kidney Liquid from Mountain States Health Products (have your licensed healthcare practitioner call 800-MHP-0074).

If a detox program isn't successfully balancing the terrain, it's often because the herbs being used are causing acid-forming reactions or overstimulating the thyroid or adrenals. Acidic urinary or salivary pH readings for more than seven days during detoxification usually indicate that the detox is too rapid or the herbs are causing an acidic reaction. Your body can't detoxify fully and properly if its pH is significantly out of whack. In this case, discontinue the detox herbs for three days and monitor your pH. If your readings go back to normal—around 6.5—try the detox herbs again, but this time add more alkalizing foods to your diet. If your pH does not normalize after that, try a different detox program or formula.

Using Supplements to Balance Your Terrain

I have found that using Juice Plus+® as a foundational nutritional supplement works to the benefit of virtually all of my clients. Juice Plus+® contains natural juice and pulp powders from fifteen different fruits and vegetables, as well as bran from two grains. The powders are concentrated using a proprietary, low-temperature process that retains as much of the foods' original nutrition as possible. As a whole-food based supplement, these powders contain a natural balance of vitamins, minerals, antioxidants, and phytonutrients. That's why Juice Plus+® is in the category of a foundational supplement that everybody can use as a baseline before adding any other supplements to their routine.

The supplements described below are suggested for use in balancing your pH and also your endocrine glands (thyroid, adrenals, and pituitary, as described in the next two chapters). These supplements can be purchased at many health food stores or from other distributors. If you choose to use them, you are unlikely to use all of them, and most of them are only taken for a short period of time as needed, until your terrain is balanced. It's a good idea, however, to learn about them, in case you ever need them for a detoxification or some other purpose.

Remember, a supplement is just that: an addition to your diet and lifestyle, not a replacement. You shouldn't rely on supplements to make up for a poor diet and unhealthy lifestyle choices.

Amino acids. Supplemental amino acids are suggested for people with highly alkaline saliva readings, as this pH indicator means they do not have enough HCl to digest protein properly and therefore may be deficient in essential amino acids. (HCl is discussed below.) As mentioned previously, vegetarians often have alkaline saliva.

Your endocrine glands cannot build their normal hormonal secretions without the proper components, and these include amino acids (as well as the right fats and trace minerals). For example, the amino acid tyrosine is needed for the thyroid to produce its hormones, and L-phenylalanine must be present for adrenal functions. That is why the ProMetabolics Terrain-Balancing Chart suggests amino acids to correct the endocrine imbalance indicated by high or low temperature or low blood pressure (discussed in the next chapter).

Sodium and potassium. Sodium and potassium are discussed in the next chapter, which also provides lists showing the sodium and potassium content of various foods. As long as you're eating natural foods and preparing your meals with your health in mind, it's easy to maintain your body's proper sodium-potassium balance.

However, if your blood pressure is low, indicating reduced adrenal activity, increase your intake of naturally sodium-rich foods, and add Celtic Sea Salt® to your diet. (Celtic Sea Salt® is described below.) You really don't have to cut back on potassium-rich foods, especially if you're on a good diet. Just don't eat a dozen bananas in one day or take a potassium supplement if you have low blood pressure.

If your blood pressure is high, cut back on unnatural sodium (refined salt) and watch out for highly salted foods, especially in restaurants. Natural foods that contain sodium should be no problem, however, and you can still use Celtic Sea Salt® to flavor your food. Meanwhile, increase your potassium intake—now you can eat those dozen bananas.

Adrenal support. Adrenal issues are detailed in the next chapter. In brief, high or low blood pressure reflects high or low adrenal activity and hormone output. For low blood pressure, the ProMetabolics Terrain-Balancing Chart suggests adrenal support such as a homeopathic formula and a whole-glandular extract, along with a few other balancing options.

If one gland is "hyper" or "hypo," the other glands can be affected, and chronic illnesses can result. A low-functioning thyroid, for example, can affect the adrenals' output of hormones. If the adrenals are already low-functioning, overloading the thyroid (with thyroid hormones, iodine, or other thyroid supplementation) can precipitate adrenal failure. I have seen low adrenal hormone levels in clients with lupus, chronic fatigue syndrome, fibromyalgia, colitis, arthritis, and cancer.

Synthetic hormones should be avoided; not only do they target a single gland, but they have an unnatural chemical structure, and the body cannot utilize them properly. Rather than using hormone replacement therapy (HRT), I have found it very effective to support and rejuvenate the glands by combining homeopathic remedies, which stimulate the body from an energic level to produce hormones, with whole-glandular extracts and other supplements, which supply the necessary nutrients.

Iodine. Our diet is often too low in iodine. When a tissue or organ becomes deficient in its dominant nutrient, either hyper- or hypo-functioning can result. That is why the ProMetabolics Terrain-Balancing Chart suggests iodine for both a high body temperature, which reflects an overactive thyroid, as well as a low body temperature, which reflects an underactive thyroid.

All bodily functions slow down when thyroid activity is reduced. Symptoms of a hypothyroid condition are "brain fog," cold hands and feet, brittle nails, dry skin, irritability, fatigue, muscle cramps, weight gain, constipation, hair loss, nervousness, panic attacks, and depression. But if a thyroid hormone is given, the body's metabolism will be stimulated, which increases the need for iodine and can actually lead to a more serious iodine deficiency. In women, the ovaries, breasts, and thyroid compete for the available iodine and respond to its deficiency by enlarging; this can cause hyperplasia in these tissues, which is a precancerous condition.

A list of iodine-rich foods is provided in the next chapter. If you choose to use an iodine supplement, a formula containing both iodine and iodide is preferable, because each form is utilized by different tissues. The breasts and prostate have high concentrations of iodine; the thyroid and skin, iodide; and the spleen, blood, and liver can have either. Such a supplement can be taken until monitoring indicates that your thyroid activity has normalized. Then you can switch to a whole-food supplement such as seaweed concentrate. (Seaweed is described below.)

Iodine is one of a group of substances called halides, which also includes bromide, chloride, and fluoride. Unfortunately, those other halides are toxins that mimic iodine by attaching themselves to your cells' iodine receptors, interfering with iodine transfer in the body. This can exacerbate a dietary iodine deficiency and throw your whole endocrine system out of balance. That's one of the reasons why it is so important to use this monitoring system to check up on your glands. (Bromide is found in bakery products, and fluoride and chloride are found in toothpaste and in our water supply. Halides are also found in various medications.)

Hydrochloric acid (HCl). Supplemental betaine hydrochloride (a form of HCl) is useful for people who cannot digest proteins properly. It also helps eliminate intestinal fermentation and limits fungal and Candida growth. Sometimes HCl and digestive enzymes are used together; a person with alkaline saliva usually needs both, as indicated by the ProMetabolics Terrain-Balancing Chart. (Enzymes are discussed below.)

People with acid reflux take over-the-counter alkalizing substances, thinking they have too much acid in their stomach, but they're mistaken—the problem is actually a lack of HCl, and the burning they feel is acid from the resulting fermentation of protein in the digestive tract. If you have acid reflux, keep your diet simple, read this book's section on food combinations, use HCl with caution, add digestive enzymes, and don't drink anything at meals but water (not too much). There's your solution.

For some people, supplemental HCl bothers the stomach. As an alternative, you can take 1 teaspoon of organic apple cider vinegar in a cup of water before meals, along with your enzyme supplement.

Enzymes. I recommend digestive enzymes to my clients for virtually every condition. Over time, your enzyme reserve is depleted by bad eating habits and years of eating cooked food in which the naturally occurring enzymes have been destroyed. Enzyme depletion can lead to inadequate digestion, resulting in nutrient deficiencies that have a detrimental effect on your internal terrain. I strongly encourage you to eat more raw foods, and I suggest taking an enzyme supplement regularly to compensate for eating cooked food, as well as to help correct any imbalances that may occur from time to time.

Supplemental digestive enzymes are especially good for people who have abnormal salivary and urinary pH readings. The ProMetabolics Terrain-Balancing Chart suggests taking enzymes for any of the six pH categories shown. Make sure your supplement contains all four digestive enzyme families: ripase, cellulase, amylase, and protease. (See the Enzymes chapter.)

Try using enzymes first for three days, and if there's no change, add HCl. You can take both at the same time if you wish, but I always prefer to test one supplement at a time. While taking HCl and digestive enzymes, eat protein foods to see whether you're now able to digest them; however, if your saliva then becomes acidic for three days in a row, this indicates that you don't need those supplements to digest protein.

The chart also suggests taking enzymes for the endocrine imbalances indicated by high or low temperature or blood pressure. There is a connection between low enzyme levels and hormone levels: if proteins and fats are not digested properly due to lack of enzymes, you can become hormone-deficient, because your endocrine glands are not receiving the nutrients they need to synthesize their hormones. If you're interested in anti-aging, take enzymes with every meal.

Celtic Sea Salt®. Refined table salt contains sodium and chloride and little else; it is a highly processed and unnatural substance. By contrast, Celtic

Sea Salt® is unrefined salt in its natural, unaltered state and contains over eighty minerals. You already know that acidity in the body is usually associated with a lack of minerals, so it's not rocket science to realize that this unrefined salt will help balance your pH by providing alkalizing organic minerals. In *Salt: Your Way to Health,* Dr. David Brownstein recounts experiments showing that half a teaspoon of Celtic Sea Salt® in a quart of water can bring the pH to normal (6.5–6.8). *(Brownstein D. Salt: Your Way to Health. Medical Alternatives Press, West Bloomfield, MI, 2006.)*

Refined table salt acidifies the body and can cause a mineral deficiency—and weight gain. Using refined salt also raises blood pressure, because the sodium is not balanced by other minerals. Unfortunately, evidence shows that a low-sodium diet does little to lower blood pressure. On a low-sodium diet, the body increases its levels of hormones such as aldosterone, rennin, angiotensin, and noradrenalin, which cause the kidneys to retain more sodium. This stimulates the sympathetic nervous system and puts the body under stress. *(Del Rio A, Rodriguez Villamil JL. Metabolic effects of strict salt restriction in essential hypertensive patients. J Intern Med 1993, 233:409-441.)*

The naturally balanced minerals in Celtic Sea Salt® can actually lower blood pressure in some cases; however, there are many clinical variables that should be evaluated by a healthcare professional before Celtic Sea Salt® is used for that purpose.

A diet particularly low in both sodium and potassium can lead to adrenal exhaustion. Decreased secretion of adrenal hormones can lead in turn to just about every disease from arthritis, fibromyalgia, and autoimmune disorders to thyroid problems.

Furthermore, elevated insulin levels have been found on low-salt diets—and you now know that elevated insulin is associated with numerous metabolic disorders, including diabetes and obesity. Dr. Brownstein states, "I have found it nearly impossible to treat insulin resistance and diabetes on a low-salt diet. Unrefined salt is a necessity when treating any condition associated with elevated insulin levels."

Although Celtic Sea Salt® contains the minerals (iodine, selenium, magnesium, and a few others) necessary for producing thyroid hormones, additional iodine may be needed in some instances. Adding seaweed to your diet may be helpful, as it is the most iodine-rich food source.

Seaweed. Seaweeds such as kelp, dulse, wakame, and nori are naturally iodine-rich foods. The ProMetabolics Terrain-Balancing Chart suggests seaweed for people with low body temperature reflecting reduced thyroid activity. It can be eaten daily as long as you don't have high blood pressure. Seaweed is a great nutritious food for everybody, as long as the body is in balance.

Green foods and juices. Most people don't eat enough green foods in their raw state; they're usually cooked, and their enzymes are destroyed. By contrast, this is why Juice Plus+® works so well. (See the Juice Plus+® chapter.) Green foods such as barley grass, chlorella, spirulina, and wheatgrass contain enzymes, chlorophyll, and magnesium, which are great for rebuilding and supporting pituitary function.

We should all eat plenty of green foods daily. The ProMetabolics Terrain-Balancing Chart suggests using green foods and juices for correcting acidic conditions and balancing thyroid and adrenal function.

Minerals. As shown on the ProMetabolics Terrain-Balancing Chart, it's good to increase your mineral intake if you have acidic saliva and/or urine—as long as your other pH reading is not alkaline. Ideally, minerals should come from food, but foods nowadays can be lacking in minerals. In some situations, particularly as you get older, you may need a mineral-rich whole-food concentrate or a supplement from a reputable company.

If monitoring shows all your readings are normal, it's okay to take a daily mineral supplement as insurance to back up mineral-deficient food.

You're almost always fighting to keep your body from acidifying out of the optimal, normal pH range, and minerals are what you need to win that fight. One formula I suggest for alkalizing the terrain is Alka C, and another is Balanced Minerals, from Innate Response; both are available through Mountain States Health Products.

The best way to take minerals, however, is in their elemental form. Elemental minerals (also called water-soluble minerals) are better utilized by the body because they are much smaller than ionic minerals and are absorbed into the bloodstream within 30–45 seconds after entering the upper stomach. Reality Health Research (877-454-3313) offers a multimineral liquid and a good calcium and magnesium liquid formula. As Dr. Lynell Braught, the creator of these products, explains: "If a mineral is too large to be absorbed into a cell, sometimes it lodges between cells. This can lead to mineral deposits."

You Can Do It: General pH Adjustment Guidelines

At first, all of this information and explanation may seem difficult to understand. But it's actually very easy to monitor your pH and to correct it, if necessary, through your food choices and by consulting the ProMetabolics Terrain-Balancing Chart for additional suggestions.

A recap of the pH categories:
- pH category 1, saliva acidic/urine alkaline – means your body is retaining acids, and liver detox may be necessary in addition to balancing pH. You may have noticeable digestive problems.

- pH category 2, saliva alkaline/urine acidic – means protein is not being digested properly, so fermentation is occurring in your intestinal tract. You may have a Candida or other fungal infection.
- pH category 3, saliva acidic/urine acidic – means your body needs alkalinity, possibly a detox program, and a change in diet. Examples of high-acid conditions are arthritis, inflammatory diseases, fibromyalgia, acid stomach, and irritable bowel syndrome.
- pH category 4, saliva alkaline/urine alkaline – means protein digestion is poor, and digestive enzymes and HCl are lacking. Examples of high-alkaline conditions are bloating and an array of digestive problems.
- pH category 5, saliva acidic/urine normal – means you may need digestive enzymes, liver detoxification, plenty of water, and probably a colon cleanse such as a series of colonics or enemas. You may have noticeable digestive and/or intestinal problems.
- pH category 6, saliva normal/urine acidic – means your kidneys may be overworked and need detoxification, so you may need a kidney-support formula, plenty of water, and possibly blood-cleansing herbs with a series of colonics.

Several important pH-balancing reminders:

- Give your body a break from taking supplements one day a week.
- If you need supplemental digestive enzymes, make sure they're plant-derived and not animal-derived pancreatic extracts. (See the Enzymes chapter; see also my book *Food Enzymes: The Missing Link to Radiant Health,* from Hohm Press.)
- If your urine or saliva is alkaline, reduce or discontinue taking minerals until you're balanced, and then slowly add them back.
- If you are acidic, do not take B-vitamins, as they have a tendency to acidify the body.

- It's best to eat fruit alone as a meal, rather than as a part of meals of other foods. Best times to eat fruit are in the morning or on hot days.
- Keep your grain consumption to sprouted and 100 percent whole-grain products. Avoid white flour and processed grain products.
- Don't drink a lot of liquid with meals, because that dilutes your digestive juices. Have just a little water or red wine at mealtime.
- If you have any chronic disorders, especially arthritis, eliminate any foods in the nightshade family, which are tobacco and its relatives such as tomatoes, eggplants, potatoes, and peppers (sweet and hot).

You may choose to work only with your salivary and urinary pH and leave it at that. Or, you may choose to go further with self-monitoring to assess and balance your endocrine system. I suggest working with pH first and getting comfortable with it, then adding thyroid monitoring, then adrenal monitoring, and then pituitary monitoring, as described in the upcoming chapters. Don't worry, prior knowledge of anatomy, nutrition, and physiology isn't required. It's all very easy—just take your time. Once you get it, you'll never regret it. Having control over your health is a wonderful thing. It's almost like controlling your future.

As I said earlier, if you've tried to balance your pH for a prolonged period and are still having trouble with it, this might indicate a chronic condition of some kind, and you should consider seeing a healthcare practitioner. (For more about pH monitoring, see www.LSMUSA.org.)

MONITORING AND SUPPORTING
THE THYROID AND ADRENAL GLANDS

Ready to add more components to your health monitoring system? The next one is body temperature, which reflects thyroid gland activity. Then comes blood pressure, which reflects adrenal gland activity. As you'll see, these glands have a close relationship.

Balancing your pH for an optimal cellular environment is obviously going to have a positive effect on your entire endocrine system. Balancing your thyroid and adrenals on top of that is a huge bonus, and can usually be achieved through dietary adjustment and taking natural supplements. If you have any concerns about your hormones, however, you should see your doctor and request the appropriate hormone panel blood tests.

Functions of the Thyroid Gland

As you may know, the trace mineral iodine is necessary for proper thyroid activity and hormone production. Iodine requires a practically perfect pH, 6.3–6.6, to be absorbed from food. This is one of the umpteen reasons why balancing your pH is so important. And conversely, monitoring your thyroid by checking your temperature will help explain why you sometimes might not be able to balance your pH.

The thyroid has numerous functions:
- maintains body temperature
- helps regulate fat metabolism
- promotes intestinal absorption of carbohydrates
- lowers cholesterol in the bloodstream
- increases urinary excretion of uric acid
- is necessary for the liver's conversion of carotene to vitamin A
- increases vessel dilation for blood and lymph circulation into cells

- reduces reflex reaction time
- is essential for normal menstrual cycles and fertility
- normalizes breast milk secretion
- attracts potassium to cells and prevents excess sodium accumulation
- keeps blood pressure below dangerous levels

Maintaining a steady body temperature is one of the thyroid's most crucial jobs. Many of the enzymes, vitamins, minerals, and chemical reactions that the body depends on are sensitive to temperature. In addition, every muscle, organ, and cell depends on thyroid hormones for optimal functioning. When the thyroid's release of hormones is inadequate to meet these demands, the body's metabolic rate is reduced, and the body is in an unhealthy state of hypothyroidism. This leads to some or all of the undesirable effects listed below.

Signs and Symptoms of Hypothyroidism

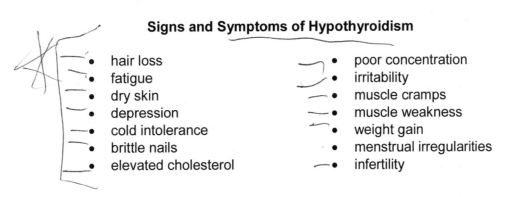

- hair loss
- fatigue
- dry skin
- depression
- cold intolerance
- brittle nails
- elevated cholesterol

- poor concentration
- irritability
- muscle cramps
- muscle weakness
- weight gain
- menstrual irregularities
- infertility

Inadequate thyroid function also causes serious problems including decreased bone marrow metabolism and decreased intestinal absorption of vitamin B_{12}; in children, it can cause mental retardation and defective myelin sheathing (insulation) around the nerves.

When the thyroid releases excessive amounts of hormones, metabolism is elevated, and the body is in an unhealthy state of hyperthyroidism. If this "hyper" condition continues, the thyroid gland will become exhausted, leading to the problems listed below.

Signs and Symptoms of Hyperthyroidism

- nervousness
- sweating
- nerve tingling
- heat intolerance
- hyperactivity

- hypertension
- weight loss
- infections
- autoimmune disorders

Thyroid problems are fairly common. It has been estimated that 30 percent of the American population has a hypothyroid condition, and I have found this to be true in my practice. Interestingly, a high percentage of fibromyalgia patients have hypothyroidism. Heavy metal toxicity has been shown to cause thyroid dysfunction, and drugs such as asthma medications, estrogens, and beta-blockers also have a disruptive effect on thyroid function.

Thyroid activity is closely interrelated with the activity of other glands, particularly the adrenals and pituitary; therefore, imbalances in thyroid hormones are highly likely to cause imbalances in the hormones of those other glands as well, including growth hormone, testosterone, progesterone, and several more.

How to Monitor Your Body Temperature

When the proper balance exists between the body's oxygen and fuel, body temperature should register in the ideal range of 98.0–99.0°F. To monitor your thyroid function, you'll be taking your temperature with an oral thermometer three times a day, at the same times that you're testing your urinary and salivary pH. If you want to get fancy, you can take your temperature hourly and time your eating of protein foods to be when your temperature is at its highest, as that's when your digestion is at its best—but that's an extra effort that you may not be interested in.

As a general guideline, it is best not to have any food less than an hour before temperature taking and not to have any liquids right before temperature taking. Please note also that after exercise or a stressful situation, you should not take a temperature reading until at least an hour has passed.

Morning temperature. Take your morning temperature while you're still in bed, before you get up to go to the bathroom (keep a thermometer by your bed). Morning temperature readings should be in the range of 97.0–98.0°. Although the morning temperature is usually lower than the midday temperature, this does not indicate a thyroid imbalance.

Midday temperature. Take your midday temperature two hours after your midday meal or snack. Midday readings should be in the normal range—no higher than 99.0°, no lower than 98.0°—and ideally, as close to 98.6° as possible.

Evening temperature. Take your evening temperature around 8:00 p.m. Evening readings should be in the range of 98.6–99.0°. Although the evening temperature is usually lower than the midday temperature, this does not indicate a thyroid imbalance.

If you are a woman of menstruating age, it's best to start your temperature monitoring period on the second day of your cycle (your menstrual cycle begins the first day after the previous cycle's bleeding has ended). During ovulation, it's natural to have an elevated temperature, which will obscure the picture if you're trying to monitor at that time.

Monitor your temperature for three to five days, and average your temperature readings for this observation period as shown in the example below.

Temperature Averaging Method

1. Calculate your average temperature at the end of each day:

> *Temperature*
> Morning   97.5
> Midday   98.2
> Evening   98.0
>   Total: 293.7

2. Divide the temperature total by the number of readings for the day's average temperature: 298.7 ÷ 3 = 97.9

3. At the end of your three- to five-day observation period, add your days' averages together and divide that total by the number of days for your final temperature average.

You can consult the ProMetabolics Terrain-Balancing Chart (shown in the previous chapter) to see what sorts of adjustments might be needed according to your temperature results.

Seaweeds and/or iodine. If you come up with an average temperature that's slightly low, below 98.0°, you can probably push it back up into the normal range by using foods and supplements that contain iodine. A list showing the iodine content of various foods is provided below. Try seaweeds such as kelp and dulse in capsule form, taken with meals. Increase the dose every seven days until you identify the best dose for you by monitoring your temperature. Some people need more than others.

Celtic Sea Salt® can also be used in this situation. (See the information on seaweeds, iodine, and Celtic Sea Salt® in the previous chapter.)

Iodine supplements are usually taken separately from meals. Reality Health Research (877-454-3313) offers iodine in elemental liquid form, and IPCS (800-838-8727) offers an excellent product called Iosol.

Iodine Content of Selected Foods
Shown in milligrams per 100-gram serving
* Asterisks indicate foods especially high in iodine

150.000	Kelp *	.020	Rutabaga	.009	Peaches, dried
8.000	Dulse *	.020	Peanuts	.009	Coconut cream
.099	Swiss chard *	.019	Strawberries *	.009	Beets
.076	Turnip greens *	.018	Artichoke (globe) *	.007	Celery
.062	Summer squash *	.017	Collard greens *	.006	Pears, dried
.043	Mustard greens *	.017	Eggplant *	.005	Cranberries
.040	Watermelon *	.016	Peaches, fresh *	.005	Lemon juice
.037	Cucumbers *	.014	Snap beans	.004	Figs
.036	Spinach *	.014	Onions (mature dry)	.004	Plums
.030	Asparagus *	.012	Bananas	.003	Broccoli
.026	Kale *	.012	Carrots	.002	Pineapple
.025	Turnip *	.010	Sweet potato	.002	Almonds
.022	Okra *	.010	Tomatoes (ripe)	.001	Grapefruit
.020	Blueberries *	.009	Apples	.001	Dates

Amino acids. You can see that the ProMetabolics Terrain-Balancing Chart suggests amino acids when temperature readings are outside of the normal range. (See the Amino Acids chapter; for more information, read Robert Erdmann's *The Amino Revolution*, published by Fireside.) Supplemental tyrosine can be taken with meals. Tyrosine is an amino acid needed by the thyroid for the manufacture of thyroxin, which is the hormone that regulates the body's growth and rate of metabolism.

Probiotics and enzymes. Sometimes when thyroid function is low, you'll see acidic pH readings. This is usually due to slow digestion, inadequate digestion of protein, or lack of digestive enzymes, any of which can set up a fermentation process in the digestive tract, leading to the body's absorption of acids from undigested food. In this case, back off meat, dairy, alcohol, grains, and coffee. Make sure your bowels are moving regularly, as it's very important to keep all of your eliminating organs working properly.

If you have poor digestion, low thyroid activity indicated by low body temperature, and an acidic salivary or urinary pH, it would be good to take probiotics and digestive enzymes, along with eating more iodine-rich foods (see the food list below) and seaweed. Probiotics are bacteria, such as *Lactobacillus acidophilus* and *Bifidobacterium bifidum,* that normally live in our bodies and contribute to our digestive process. Unfortunately, we often disrupt our internal environment by destroying our own helpful bacteria, usually thanks to coffee, high protein, high sugar, low fiber, stress, antibiotics, altered pH, or lack of digestive enzymes. (Probiotics are discussed in the chapter on Choosing the Right Diet and Supplements.)

Green foods and juices. The ProMetabolics Terrain-Balancing Chart also suggests green foods and juices for both high and low temperature. These are foundational nutrition for thyroid problems. Green foods and juices contain a variety of thyroid-supportive minerals, are cooling for the body, and help with any pH imbalance. They also help with detoxification, especially concentrated green powders.

Glandular products. If your average temperature is very low, around 96.5–97.0°, you may need to take a different approach. You may wish to consult a nutritionist about using a glandular product for low thyroid function. A whole-glandular is a concentrated extract derived from the glands of certain animals. Your body will digest this extract and your glands will use whatever components they need.

Glandulars should only be used sparingly and in conjunction with other nutritional support. Whole-glandular products typically contain substances that the glands need to start producing on their own again, so they should not be taken for more than one to two months. That is why it's good to use homeopathic formulas along with glandulars, because the homeopathics stimulate the gland in question to become active and work on its own until it doesn't need the glandular raw materials anymore. You can then continue taking the homeopathic formula until your monitoring shows that the gland is balanced.

Caution: If you have high blood pressure, you should not use animal-derived whole adrenal glandulars. They often contain adrenaline, which can over-stimulate your adrenals, thyroid, or pituitary. If any of your glands are hyperactive, don't take a glandular product unless that specific hormone has been removed from it.

Armour Thyroid is a desiccated porcine thyroid glandular available by prescription. (It is highly recommended in Dr. David Brownstein's book *Overcoming Thyroid Disorders,* from Medical Alternatives Press.) However, this product should be avoided by anyone who can't tolerate corn starch, which is an ingredient in the formula. Some glandulars I recommend are Thyroid Support and Thyroid Glandular from Mountain States Health Products (have your licensed healthcare practitioner call 800-MHP-0074). These products are derived from animals raised in New Zealand that are free of the disease bovine spongiform encephalopathy (BSE) and range-fed, and the formulas include enzymes for better utilization by the body. Mountain States also offers homeopathic remedies, Thyroid Liquid and Thyroid Drops, for balancing thyroid function.

A note about hyperthyroidism. Elevated temperature readings of 100° or higher can be indicative of hyperthyroidism and may be accompanied by other symptoms such as nervousness, hyperactivity, mental confusion, or even extreme temper, and possibly a rapid pulse (see the Pituitary chapter). Hyperthyroidism is not often mentioned in self-help books because it's not a common condition.

Although this may seem strange, you can usually use the same methods to correct hyperthyroidism as those described above for hypothyroidism. In hyperthyroidism, the thyroid is working very hard, possibly because it does not have enough iodine or tyrosine to make its hormones; this condition can lead to hypertrophy (enlargement) of the gland. But the same deficiency can also lead to hypothyroidism, which similarly indicates an overworked thyroid. Hyper can also lead to hypo, and either of these conditions can be related to a long-term infection as well. Once your pH is corrected and your blood pressure is also normal, hyperthyroidism usually balances out. But if you cannot balance your thyroid, you should see a healthcare practitioner.

Blood Pressure and Your Adrenal Glands

Your blood pressure gives you information on how your adrenal glands are functioning. The adrenal glands sit on top of the kidneys, in the lower back. Often, lower back pain is caused by adrenal exhaustion. The adrenals produce the "fight-or-flight" hormones, adrenaline and cortisol, that prepare the body for stressful situations, as well as the steroid hormones that help the body fight infections, heal injuries, and regulate blood sugar. Cortisol is secreted under conditions of stress, injury, and infection; it helps regulate blood sugar and makes amino acids available for use.

The adrenals also produce sex hormones: dehydroepiandrosterone (DHEA), pregnenolone, testosterone, estrogen, and progesterone are all manufactured in the adrenals of both men and women. In women, though, estrogen and progesterone are primarily produced by the ovaries until menopause, and then the adrenals become the major estrogen source. This is why so many people in their forties and fifties need hormone replacement therapy (HRT). Toxicity, nutritional imbalances, and glandular deficiencies can be the cause.

As noted, there is a close interrelationship between the thyroid and adrenal glands and their respective hormones, so it's important to balance both the thyroid and adrenals. Allergies, asthma, depression, anxiety, ulcerative colitis, hypertension, cancer, chronic fatigue syndrome, and fibromyalgia are all indicators of endocrine imbalance—such as hypothyroidism and/or hypoadrenalism—because the two glands work synergistically. For instance, in a hypothyroid state, the body's adrenal hydrocortisone level has been found to be low. Research has also shown a close relationship between low DHEA levels and low thyroid hormone levels. One gland's weakness over a long period of time can weaken the other. We often see both glands in a low-functioning "hypo" state during chronic illness.

I suggest that if you suspect thyroid or adrenal issues, the first thing to do is to look at all your readings—saliva, urine, blood pressure, temperature—and, as long as you're not in an emergency situation, try to balance them with good nutrition (see Part Four of this book). The second thing to do is have blood work done to check your adrenal, thyroid, and growth hormones.

Using the ProMetabolics monitoring system goes a long way toward balancing the endocrine system with the raw materials that your glands need to produce their hormones as they should. If all else fails, find a physician who does HRT. One treatment option is to find a compounding pharmacy to make you a perfectly balanced, custom-made hormonal cream. Then every three months, get your hormonal blood analysis done, but always continue your monitoring system. An excellent compounding pharmacy that I use is Bert's Pharmacy, a wonderful, family-owned pharmacy in Sayre, PA (570-888-2157).

How to Monitor Your Blood Pressure

You can purchase a home blood pressure monitor at any drugstore, or take your blood pressure right there if the store has a public machine that you can use. Either way, follow the instructions carefully. A home monitor is not too expensive and it's worth purchasing if you're going to monitor your blood pressure regularly.

Unlike your other readings, you only need to take this once during the day. I usually suggest taking a blood pressure reading once every three to five days, but you can take it every day if you wish. For a good indication of your day's blood pressure, the best times to take it are 10:00 a.m. or 2:00–3:00 p.m. Don't take a reading after exercise or exertion, until at least an hour has passed. If you check your blood pressure every day for a three- to five-day monitoring period, average the readings as you do with your pH and temperature.

Normal systolic and diastolic pressure. When you take your blood pressure, you actually take two measurements, which are written like a fraction: the top number is systolic pressure, which is the pressure during the heart's beat, and the bottom is diastolic pressure, which is the pressure between beats. This is the normal range for those two measurements:

systolic	110–135
diastolic	65–85

Interpreting your blood pressure numbers. Let's say you've taken your blood pressure measurement and it's 140/90. Add your systolic and diastolic numbers together: 140 + 90 = 230. Divide the total by 2: 230/2 = 115. That final number, in this case 115, is the one you'll look at for the purposes of the monitoring system. If the number you reach by this method is 90 or lower, your blood pressure is low. If it is 110 or higher, your blood pressure is high.

Another easy, quick test of your adrenal status is to take your blood pressure lying down, and then immediately stand up and take it again. It should go up five to ten points—if it does not, this indicates low adrenal function.

Blood Pressure, Sodium, and Potassium

Blood pressure is strongly affected by the balance between sodium and potassium, because the amounts of these two minerals in the body are directly related to adrenal function. No doubt you've heard that people who have high blood pressure should lower their sodium intake. Well, nobody should use ordinary refined table salt, regardless of their blood pressure, because it lacks minerals (aside from sodium, of course) and acidifies the body, particularly the digestive tract. (See the discussion of Celtic Sea Salt® in the previous chapter.)

Overactive adrenals make your cells hold on to more sodium while letting your kidneys excrete more potassium. The sodium makes cells and vessels contract, and as the adrenals continue to be hyper, blood pressure goes up. If you have low blood pressure, the opposite is happening—that is, underactive adrenals are leading to excretion of sodium and retention of potassium. By adjusting your dietary intake of one or both of these minerals, you can adjust your blood pressure. Lists of the sodium and potassium content in various foods are provided below.

Supporting Exhausted Adrenal Glands

One of the reasons why it is good to look at all of the monitoring system's readings together is that trying to balance your pH without addressing any glandular problem that may be present can be difficult or even impossible—and vice versa. For example, if your blood pressure is high, your adrenals are being overworked, which can cause over-acidity and inflammation. Always look deeper into the imbalance if you find that you can't correct your pH with dietary adjustments alone.

To support and balance your adrenals, first nourish them through your diet for one to two weeks before turning to supplements. If you don't see an improvement, refer to the ProMetabolics Terrain-Balancing Chart and the list below for suggested supplements. Try one at a time; give it one week, and monitor its effect.

Vitamins and herbs. Specific nutrients needed by the adrenals are vitamin C (take it in ascorbate form, not ascorbic acid), pantothenic acid, and zinc. A B-complex supplement that includes pantothenic acid is good for the adrenals as long as the body is not acidic (B-vitamins can be acidifying).

Licorice root (do not use licorice if you have high blood pressure), Siberian ginseng (*Eleutheroccocus senticosus*), Chinese ginseng (*Panax ginseng*), gotu kola, and ashwagandha are good herbs for the adrenals. (See the chapter on Choosing the Right Diet and Supplements.) Your health food store will have herbal combinations for adrenals. Gaia Herbs and Herb Pharm are two reputable online sources for herbal products. Mountain States Health Products also offers many herb-based combinations that help support adrenal function (800-MHP-0074).

Amino acids. The amino acid phenylalanine is very important for the production of adrenaline and also for a group of neurotransmitters or "brain hormones" called catecholamines. When catecholamine levels are normal, they contribute to alertness and help the body respond to stress. Another action of phenylalanine is to stimulate the intestines to produce a hormone called cholecystokinin, which signals the brain that you have eaten enough food. Taken together, supplemental phenylalanine and tyrosine improve your production of adrenal and thyroid hormones. (See the Amino Acids chapter.)

The ProMetabolics Terrain-Balancing Chart suggests using amino acids when your blood pressure readings are low. Do not use them, however, if you have high blood pressure.

Sodium and potassium. The ProMetabolics Terrain-Balancing Chart suggests decreasing sodium and increasing potassium if your blood pressure is high, and increasing sodium if your blood pressure is low. See the food lists below. Remember, ordinary table salt is no good for anybody; use Celtic Sea Salt® instead.

For high blood pressure, you can also take a potassium supplement in the form of potassium gluconate, potassium bicarbonate, potassium phosphate, or potassium acetate. Potassium is part of your buffering system and will help alkalize your pH. Potassium pushes sodium out of the cells. (That's why body-builders use potassium to help shed extra water-weight before a contest.)

Sodium Content of Selected Foods
Shown in milligrams per 100-gram serving

3,007	Kelp	18	Radishes
2,892	Irish moss	16	Peach
2,400	Olives	15	Cashew
2,085	Dulse	15	Broccoli
147	Swiss chard	14	Brussels sprouts
130	Beet greens	14	Endive
126	Celery	13	Cauliflower
76	Dandelion	13	Green pepper
75	Kale	12	Cantaloupe
71	Spinach	12	Honeydew
60	Beets	12	Parsnips
52	Watercress	10	Sweet potato
47	Carrot	9	Brown rice
45	Parsley	8	Prunes
49	Turnips	8	Horseradish
43	Artichoke	8	Kohlrabi
43	Collard greens	7	Mango
35	Cow peas	7	Snap peas
34	Fig	6	Cucumber
30	Lentils	5	Plantain
27	Raisins	5	Leeks
26	Apricot	5	Onions
26	Red cabbage	4	Avocado
26	Chick pea	4	Almonds
25	Coconut	4	Lima beans
22	Savoy cabbage	3	Okra
19	Garlic	3	Potato skin
19	White beans	3	Tomatoes

Potassium Content of Selected Foods
Shown in milligrams per 100-gram serving

8,060	Dulse	529	Garlic
5,273	Kelp	470	Spinach
1,529	Lima beans	467	Rye
1,495	Rice bran	460	Walnuts
1,477	Banana	430	Millet
1,201	Hot red peppers	414	Mushrooms
1,196	White beans	407	Potato skins
1,028	Mung beans	401	Collard greens
1,979	Apricot	397	Dandelion greens
950	Peach	397	Fennel
940	Prune	390	Brussels sprouts
920	Sunflower seeds	382	Broccoli
827	Wheat germ	378	Kale
797	Chickpeas	377	Mustard greens
790	Lentils	372	Black currant
773	Almonds	372	Kohlrabi
763	Raisins	347	Leeks
727	Parsley	369	Winter squash
725	Sesame seeds	341	Carrot
648	Dates	341	Celery
640	Figs	340	Pumpkin seeds
606	Watercress	295	Cauliflower
604	Avocado	294	Endive
600	Yam	335	Beets
570	Beet greens	296	Barley
550	Swiss chard	310	Persimmon
541	Cow peas		

Enzymes and fatty acids. The ProMetabolics Terrain-Balancing Chart suggests enzymes for both high and low blood pressure. When digestion is poor, the necessary nutrients are not available to the adrenal glands, which is the root of a lot of adrenal problems, and that's why enzymes are helpful for balancing adrenal activity. That is also why it's good to supplement the body's essential fatty acids (EFAs) in either hyper or hypo gland conditions. I recommend the combined EFA formula Omega Nutrition 3-6-9 from Mountain States Health Products.

Green foods and juices. Green foods and juices are helpful for balancing adrenal activity whether your blood pressure is high or low. They are always alkalizing (hyper adrenals can produce a lot of acidity) and also very cleansing. As noted above, glandular imbalance often occurs when the body is not digesting food properly; concentrated green powders and juices are especially good in this case because they are a predigested food form that is quickly assimilated by the body for rapid pH correction and nutritional support to the glands.

Glandular products. Exhaust other methods of adrenal assistance first before trying a glandular product. Work with a nutritionist when using glandulars for low adrenal function. As mentioned earlier, glandulars should be used for no more than one or two months and in conjunction with other nutritional support. Using homeopathic formulas as well stimulates the gland in question to work on its own until it doesn't need the glandular raw materials anymore. You can then continue the homeopathic formula until monitoring shows the gland is balanced.

Caution: If you have high blood pressure, you should not use animal-derived whole adrenal glandulars. They often contain adrenaline, which can over-stimulate your adrenals, thyroid, or pituitary. If any of your glands are hyperactive, don't take a glandular product unless that specific hormone has been removed from it.

I recommend Adrenal Support from Mountain States Health Products (have your licensed healthcare practitioner call them). It is derived from animals raised in New Zealand that are free of the disease bovine spongiform encephalopathy (BSE) and range-fed, and the formula includes enzymes for better utilization by the body.

Fast Burners, Slow Burners, and Sugar

Once your endocrine system is balanced, and your pH is 6.5–6.8 for saliva and urine, you can identify whether you are a "fast burner" or a "slow burner," metabolically speaking, by experimenting with foods to determine how the different food groups affect you. If, when you increase your intake of protein and fat, your pH and endocrine status remain balanced, you're probably a fast burner who can handle these heavy foods. But if your pH turns acid from increasing protein and fat, you might want to try switching to a higher-carbohydrate diet instead— making sure to emphasize vegetable-based carbs. If further monitoring shows that this diet works better for you, you're probably a slow burner who doesn't need as much protein and fat.

The chart below shows the usual relationship between the state of your glands and the level of sugar in your body. This indicates when to eat— and when to avoid—fruits and other high-sugar foods. Example: If your temperature and blood pressure are high, indicating overactive thyroid and adrenals (the bottom row of the chart), it's likely your sugar level is high, so don't eat fruit or sugar during that time; you'd only be "feeding the heat" with more sugar and its resulting fermentation in your body.

Thyroid and Adrenal Function:

Relationship with Sugar Levels

	High sugar level	Low sugar level
Thyroid underactive Adrenals normal		X
Thyroid overactive Adrenals normal	X	
Thyroid normal Adrenals underactive		X
Thyroid normal Adrenals overactive	X	
Thyroid overactive Adrenals overactive	X	

Natural Treatment Suggestions for Cardiovascular Disease

If you suspect that you may have cardiovascular disease, please see a licensed healthcare practitioner.

Any time any sign of cardiovascular disease is present, keep your diet low in refined carbohydrates. Eat mostly raw vegetables and fruits and drink a lot of purified water. If you must cook your vegetables, steam them lightly. Eat lean meats, fish, and raw seeds and nuts (soak the seeds and nuts overnight in water to release their enzyme inhibitors). Eliminate processed baked goods, coffee, sugar, fried foods, and dairy. Keep grains at a minimum, eating only 100 percent whole grains and sprouted grains.

When you see a high systolic pressure and a low diastolic pressure, such as 140/65, plaque may be building up in your arteries. For this situation, take an iodine supplement to support the thyroid and eat whole foods to obtain all of their synergistic nutrients in proper balance. Use only the good fats: primrose oil, pumpkin seed oil, flaxseed oil, organic extra-virgin coconut oil, and sunflower oil. (See the Fats chapter.) We can all use these oils daily to prevent blood cell clumping, restore damaged cell membranes, and carry oxygen throughout the body. One suggestion is to take 1 tablespoon of flaxseed oil daily and 500 milligrams of niacin (in the form of inositol hexaniacinate) three times daily.

To prevent plaque formation and stop lipid peroxidation, vitamin E with tocotrienols is good, along with fresh garlic or "odorless garlic," vitamin C, and niacin. An extract from the mukul myrrh tree, gugulipid, has been shown in several clinical studies to lower blood lipid levels and reduce pre-existing atherosclerotic (artery-clogging and artery-hardening) plaque. Gugulipid extract containing 25 milligrams of the active ingredient guggulsterone per 500-milligram tablet, taken three times per day, is an effective dose. (See the Free Radicals and Antioxidants chapter.)

Co-enzyme Q-10, L-carnitine, hawthorn berries, and cayenne pepper are also good for most heart and arterial conditions. (See the chapter on Choosing the Right Diet and Supplements.) Aconite, Cactus, Spigelia, Lachesis, and Crataegus are a few homeopathic remedies to look into for heart afflictions. Celtic Sea Salt® can be used in all circulatory conditions. Exercise one hour daily, out in the fresh air if possible.

MONITORING AND SUPPORTING THE PITUITARY GLAND

One gland affects another through the production and release of hormones, which are involved in controlling functions beyond the gland that secreted them. Our endocrine system controls our digestive, circulatory, and nervous systems and regulates internal activities right down to cellular metabolism. When you can't balance your readings, you must look to the pituitary gland. The pituitary is often called the master gland because it secretes hormones that control thyroid and adrenal activity. If the pituitary gland is not too exhausted, too deficient in hormone materials, or too badly affected by heavy metal toxicity, you may be able to balance it by balancing thyroid activity (observed through body temperature) and adrenal activity (observed through blood pressure). A pituitary problem is usually due to imbalances in these other glands.

Chronic conditions such as cancer, diabetes, arthritis, fibromyalgia, hypoadrenalism, thyroid disease, premenstrual syndrome (PMS), and lupus are all related to imbalances in the body's terrain and hormonal system. Disease starts in the terrain and works its way up into the systems of the body. By eliminating toxins and bringing in whole foods and supplements, you enable vital nutrients to work their way up that ladder too, to support the affected systems. You can see how foolish it is to merely take a drug and not balance your terrain. If you do need to take a drug, work the monitoring system to its maximum so you may be able to get off the drug. You are ultimately responsible for your own health.

The Master Gland and Its Subjects

The pituitary gland secretes hormones that regulate the growth of all of your tissues, the secretion of some sex hormones, the secretion of the thyroid hormone thyroxin, and the secretion of several adrenal hormones—

so you can see how far-reaching the pituitary's influence is. You don't need to memorize the names of all these hormones; I'm just showing you all the connections to help you understand what you're balancing by using the monitoring system.

The Pituitary Control Factors

```
                        Pituitary
                       ↙        ↘
           Thyrotropin              ACTH
          ↙                              ↘
   Thyroid                                 Adrenals
```

Growth hormone from the pituitary promotes protein synthesis, thereby increasing the size of cellular structures throughout the body. As you age, your production of growth hormone decreases. Another pituitary product, gonadotropic hormone, controls the adrenals' secretion of sex hormones such as testosterone, estrogen, and progesterone. When a body-builder takes growth hormone, it overstimulates the pituitary, which releases gonadotropic hormone to instruct the adrenals to secrete more testosterone, leading to rapid muscle growth.

Thyrotropin from the pituitary controls the thyroid's secretion of thyroxin. When thyrotropin is deficient, the thyroid becomes incapacitated; body temperature falls and cellular metabolism decreases, which manifests as fatigue and lethargy. But taking stimulating herbs or drugs without providing the right foods for your glands only amounts to beating a dead horse. For the thyroid to produce its hormones, the amino acid tyrosine and the mineral iodine must be available in the blood.

As noted in the previous chapter, thyroxin has numerous functions, starting with controlling the cellular metabolic rate. It causes the body to burn carbohydrates rapidly and then to burn fats. A person who has excess thyroxin loses weight rapidly; a person who has too little thyroxin often develops obesity. Thyroxin also excites the nervous system, which becomes sluggish when thyroxin is diminished. In addition, thyroxin increases the gastrointestinal tract's motility (that is, its ability to move food along) and promotes the flow of digestive juices—too much thyroxin can lead to diarrhea, and too little to constipation.

A fourth pituitary product is adrenocorticotropic hormone (ACTH), which further influences the adrenal glands' hormonal output. You're probably familiar with adrenaline, also called epinephrine, and its partner norepinephrine, which stimulate the sympathetic nervous system. Other adrenal hormones called mineralocorticoids control mineral balances in the body; for example, they regulate retention of sodium by the kidneys to control the sodium-potassium balance. Mineralocorticoids also regulate some aspects of carbohydrate, fat, and protein metabolism.

Yet another group of adrenal hormones, glucocorticoids, affect the metabolism of protein, fat, and glucose. For our purposes, the most important glucocorticoid is cortisol, which is secreted under stress or during exercise. By depressing the tissues' utilization of glucose, cortisol increases the concentration of glucose in the bloodstream so the sugar can be utilized for energy as the "emergency" requires. Secondly, it causes the liver to convert proteins into more glucose.

So if you're under stress, using false stimulants such as coffee, and adding a high-carbohydrate, high-sugar diet on top of this, you can see why type II diabetes is becoming an epidemic. It is because the adrenal overstimulation from these stressors raises cortisol levels, so the bloodstream then contains too much glucose from both the body and the diet, and the pancreas can't put out enough insulin to keep up with all the blood sugar. (The Insulin chapter explains how the pancreas gets overworked and exhausted with all this sugar.)

Signs of a Possible Pituitary Problem

We age rapidly by constantly beating up our glands. Disturbed emotions such as anger burn out the thyroid and adrenals, and we feed them second-class foods full of chemicals, and then we just can't seem to figure out what causes disease—well, *we* cause disease. I've experienced gland exhaustion by pushing myself too far, and I'd like to keep you from making the same mistake.

In most situations of apparent gland imbalance or exhaustion, I suggest addressing the thyroid and adrenals first; you can usually balance them without needing to address the pituitary directly. If your body temperature and/or blood pressure is low, first try to improve your thyroid and/or adrenal function. Then, if thirty days go by and they're not responding to anything you try, that's an indication that the pituitary needs support. A situation I don't see too often is when both temperature and blood pressure remain high for a period of time (sometimes this indicates infection). An iodine-containing formula will usually rebalance those readings, but if not, turn to pituitary support. And if a chronic condition is present, you'll probably have to go after the master gland.

The Pulse and the Pituitary Gland

Your pulse can serve as another indicator of your terrain's status, as it is affected by your glands and pH. Take your pulse for 15 seconds, multiply that number by 4, and you'll get how many times it beats per minute. A normal pulse is in the range of 65–80 beats per minute. Sometimes an athlete's pulse rate may be a little lower, but 60 or less is too low. (We have all heard of athletes who have an enlarged heart with a low pulse.) If you find that your pulse rate is high or low, that's a cue to take a look at your other readings. A particular indication that your pituitary gland may be in trouble is when you see a low pulse rate along with low temperature and low blood pressure.

Supporting the Pituitary Gland and Its Partners

Chlorophyll and green juice. First try drinking liquid chlorophyll or green vegetable juices. All green embryonic dried grass juices are helpful because the natural magnesium is excellent for the pituitary. A few examples are barley juice powder, spirulina, blue-green algae, chlorella, and alfalfa. Chlorophyll is almost identical to hemoglobin, the only difference being that the chlorophyll molecule contains magnesium whereas the hemoglobin molecule contains iron. The body, however, can create hemoglobin for its red blood cells from chlorophyll. The nucleic acids, amino acids, and minerals, plus supplemental magnesium—all supplied by chlorophyll, green juice, and blue-green algae—will support the pituitary. If you use these and balance the rest of your terrain, that may take care of any pituitary problem.

Amino acids. All of your hormones, neurotransmitters, and tissues must utilize free-form amino acids to conduct their proper functions in the body. For this reason, amino acid supplementation is very helpful when trying to balance your endocrine activity; essential fatty acids are important for this purpose as well. A supplement that contains all the essential amino acids (phenylalanine, tryptophan, methionine, lysine, leucine, isoleucine, valine, and threonine) should be available at your local health food store. I like Aminoplex from Cardiovascular Formulas, distributed by Mountain States Health Products (800-MHP-0074). (See the Amino Acids chapter.)

Gland-supporting formulas and glandular products. As mentioned, pituitary support often entails supporting the thyroid and adrenal glands at the same time. Two companies offering reliable products to help balance the pituitary, thyroid, and adrenals are Standard Process (800-558-8740) and Moss Nutrition (800-851-5444). Pituitropin PMG from Standard Process is excellent. Moss offers BioThyro and Potassium Iodine for the thyroid and Adrenal Support Plus and Bio Adaptogen for the adrenals.

Whole-gland extracts must be ordered by a chiropractor, nutritionist, physician, or other licensed health professional. If you do use a glandular, it's usually best to use one that contains gland tissue but not the gland's hormones. Mountain States Health Products formulates glandulars from New Zealand animals that are free of the disease bovine spongiform encephalopathy (BSE) and range-fed. Their formulas include enzymes to enhance absorption. Mountain States also distributes herbal and vitamin-based endocrine-supporting products from Innate, Professional Solutions, and New Mark.

When using any whole-glandular supplement for pituitary, thyroid, or adrenal support, take it only for one to two months, along with other nutritional support. As previously noted, it's good to use homeopathic formulas along with glandulars, to stimulate the gland in question to become active and work on its own until it doesn't need the glandular raw materials anymore. You can then continue taking the homeopathic formula until your monitoring shows that the gland is balanced.

Caution: If you have high blood pressure, you should not use animal-derived whole adrenal glandulars. They often contain adrenaline, which can over-stimulate your adrenals, thyroid, or pituitary. If any of your glands are hyperactive, don't take a glandular product unless that specific hormone has been removed from it.

A good kinesiologist or a health practitioner who uses vibrational medicine will be able to determine which product is best for you. Your physician may also be able to recommend something that will work for you. By using the monitoring system, you can see how any treatment is affecting you. I suggest monitoring a product for a month before deciding whether or not it's effective for you.

PART THREE

ProMetabolics: Cleansing and Optimizing Body Systems

FAMILIAR DRUGS AND THEIR SIDE EFFECTS: INFLAMMATORY BOWEL, CHRONIC FATIGUE, AND FIBROMYALGIA

In this book, I've discussed that there can be many causes of any one disease. To put yourself on the road to recovery, you can start eliminating the causes of disease by making lifestyle and dietary changes. No matter what the condition is, balancing your pH and cleansing your terrain are of primary importance. Finding the core problem or focus of any disease always entails investigation, sometimes with the help of the appropriate clinical tests: blood test, urine test, fatty acid analysis, or any number of others. You might have to find a physician who uses specific diagnostic techniques. Through knowledge, you can be your own doctor. By that, I don't mean that you don't need a doctor—just that you can do many things to monitor your own health, to see where you stand at any given point in time before disease strikes. Then you can make appropriate adjustments and prevent illness. In most cases, what you do for yourself has more of an effect on your health than any other factor.

For over five decades, non-steroidal anti-inflammatory drugs (NSAIDs) have been used for inflammatory disease. These include over-the-counter drugs such as Aleve, Motrin, and Advil. Prescription NSAIDs include Indocin, Celebrex, Toradol, Feldene, and many more. In his book *Overcoming Arthritis*, Dr. David Brownstein states, "In my experience, the results of these drug therapies are dismal." (*Brownstein D. Overcoming Arthritis. Medical Alternatives Press, West Bloomfield, MI, 2001.*) These drugs may temporarily alleviate symptoms, but they do little to halt or reverse the progression of arthritic disorders. In fact, NSAIDs can suppress the endocrine system and actually inhibit the body's natural formation of cartilage. Worse, it is estimated that 16,500 patients with rheumatoid arthritis or osteoarthritis die annually from toxic effects of NSAIDs—a total similar to the number of annual deaths from AIDS.

In 1940, the discovery of cortisone for treating arthritis and other inflammatory conditions seemed like a miracle. But within a short time, adverse effects from this drug began to be reported: cataracts, hypertension, diabetes, and osteoporosis. This is another example of a treatment getting further away from the true cause of the disease it was meant to cure. Without understanding what's really behind autoimmune diseases, the layperson believes that drugs such as NSAIDs are actually curing something. Instead, drugs can inhibit natural immunity, create an acidic condition, and lead to other chronic conditions if not properly monitored.

Most people who come to see me don't even know much about the drugs they're taking or how long they should take them, and they're too afraid to ask their doctors about side effects. How can someone in this situation reverse a chronic illness? That is one of the reasons why so many diseases are seen as being chronic and incurable. When I explain that disease can be reversed and bodies brought back to normal balance, many of my clients are disbelieving because of their limited knowledge of the disease process.

By now, we have become conditioned to think that if we take a pill we're going to get better, so the idea of having to do any work at all for our own health is just too much to fathom. When NSAIDs were introduced, they were hailed for their fast action. We could buy them over the counter and get quick relief without changing our diet or lifestyle. But NSAIDs are addicting, because they break the pain cycle and patients get (temporary) relief, only to find that they need to take more of the drug as time goes on. Furthermore, NSAIDs have many side effects including kidney and liver damage, osteoporosis, irritable bowel syndrome, and leaky gut syndrome.

Many illnesses have related symptoms, and many illnesses are found in combination with each other. Chronic fatigue, hypothyroid problems, leaky gut, and fibromyalgia can all be related. This should remind you that disease is a process and not just a group of symptoms. Different diseases can have similar causes, which means once you eliminate the cause, then not only several symptoms but several different conditions can disappear at the same time.

One disease caused by a drug can lead to another disease. As an example, taking birth control pills, or taking Premarin for estrogen therapy, can increase levels of a protein called thyroxin binding globulin, which decreases the level of the thyroid hormone thyroxin. Chemotherapy also decreases thyroid output. What do the resulting symptoms resemble? Chronic fatigue syndrome. If chronic fatigue is present, there are usually digestive disturbances, and then mineral deficiencies, terrain imbalance, and adrenal fatigue. Becoming mineral-deficient affects the body's pH balance, leading to an acidic condition and pain and then to fibromyalgia. Dr. John Lowe states that 63 percent of individuals diagnosed with fibromyalgia have laboratory signs of hypothyroidism. *(Lowe JC. Thyroid status of 38 fibromyalgia patients: implications for the etiology of fibromyalgia. Clin Bull Myofasc Ther 1997 2:47-64.)*

Some of these processes get started with an environmental toxin. For instance, the fluoride in tap water is similar to iodine; consequently, it can mimic iodine in the body, which causes the thyroid to mistakenly reduce its uptake of the actual iodine that it needs. An iodine-deficient thyroid cannot make sufficient thyroid hormones. Heavy metals such as accumulated mercury or cadmium can also affect the secretion of thyroid and adrenal hormones. Stress is another factor that can deplete the adrenals through over-secretion of their hormones, leading to fatigue and immune irregularities. One of these excessively secreted adrenal hormones is cortisol, which can deplete your minerals and cause excessive insulin secretion and weight gain. One thing affects another that affects another in your body's interconnected systems.

A look at the domino effect of some of these drugs in combination with other factors will illustrate how the resulting symptoms are only reactions on the surface of a deeper cause. One effect of heavy metals, drugs such as NSAIDs, and chemicals such as pesticides is to erode the lining of the intestine, eventually creating holes, which is called leaky gut syndrome. At the same time, the combination of a poor diet and exposure to these foreign substances creates an over-acidic condition, which is a perfect environment for fungus—remember how the endobiant evolves through the bacterial stage to the fungal stage?

Now two processes are taking place at the same time, confusing the symptom picture. Fungus (including yeast) interferes with digestion, causing nutritional deficiencies and adrenal and thyroid fatigue, and it also produces waste products called mycotoxins, which further acidify the internal environment and promote additional fungal growth. The more overgrowth, the more deficiencies. Enzymes cannot function properly in this toxic, pH-imbalanced terrain, and B-vitamin deficiencies and hormonal imbalances develop. The leaky gut allows undesirable substances to be absorbed into the body through the intestinal wall, enabling fungus to set up shop in the pancreas, liver, and spleen.

Mycotoxins poison the body and trigger an immune system response. When the immune system becomes overtaxed, the result is allergic reactions to foods, chemicals, and airborne substances (discussed more below). Mycotoxins can weaken any part of the body and are a major player in ear infections, vaginal infections, rectal itch, post-nasal drip, hives, ringworm, and all mucus conditions; diaper rash, thrush, eczema, urinary tract infections, and chronic fatigue; respiratory illnesses including bronchitis and asthma; and inflammatory joint diseases such as arthritis, muscle-tendon inflammation, and fibromyalgia.

It is very difficult for the damaged, inflamed gut lining to absorb minerals and other nutrients during digestion, as it cannot produce its usual carrier proteins that deliver minerals to the bloodstream. The leaky gut also allows toxins from various sources to be absorbed into the bloodstream and dispersed through the body, damaging the energy-producing mitochondria within cells. The result? Chronic fatigue.

These poisons also go to the muscles and cause fibromyalgia, which is a condition characterized by stiffness and pain in muscles, ligaments, shoulders, hips, and connective tissues throughout the body. At this point, why would you dump an antibiotic into the mix, trying to kill bacteria or yeast, when you'd only be creating a more toxic internal environment that promotes their growth instead?

A major problem is that this disease process started in the intestines, where half of the body's detoxification capabilities reside. As intestinal inflammation becomes progressively worse, further detoxification capabilities are lost. But this is far from the end of the damage.

As undigested food particles pass through the leaky gut into the bloodstream, the immune system identifies them as invaders, or antigens, and begins to attack. White blood cells produce antibodies (also called immunoglobulins) that target, attach to, and break down these particles. The problem is that antibodies cannot always distinguish between the antigens and your body tissues—so they may begin to attack the body. The antigen-antibody complexes that are formed in this attack are a major contributing factor to arthritis, especially if the immune system is attacking the cartilage in the joints. Among the many autoimmune disorders—conditions in which the body mistakenly attacks itself—are lupus, rheumatoid arthritis, diabetes, and multiple sclerosis (MS).

This is also a way that food allergies develop. Your immune system has manufactured antibodies against the undigested particles of a particular food that it identified as an antigen, so when you eat that same food again later, your immune system responds to it with an allergic reaction: you sneeze, ache, your joints hurt, and—here's a big one that many people don't know—you experience mood disorders. Food allergies are never cured by allergy shots because the shots only address the symptoms, not the cause.

In short, drug treatment can negatively affect many parts of your body, particularly your glands and digestive tract. Some people don't realize the harm that many medications can do, and they keep turning to drug therapy whenever they're sick. But by using natural therapeutics along with any drug therapy, supporting and nourishing the body, and detoxifying properly, you can then wean yourself off drugs under a doctor's care. Both types of therapy can work together for your greater good. And by using the monitoring system during this process, you can see how medications and other treatments are affecting your terrain.

Proper digestion, and the intestinal tract itself, are so very important to our health. Most people don't know that the gut not only houses half of our detoxification mechanisms, but also half of the immune system. The whole scenario described above—the relationship between leaky gut syndrome, chronic fatigue, fibromyalgia, autoimmune diseases food allergy, and mood disorders such as anxiety and depression—demonstrates once again that disease is a process and that many diseases can be related at their root cause. This is why we must find the core or focus of a disease in order to treat it correctly. It also shows that a simple original focus—a damaged, inflamed gut wall—can produce pretty complicated symptomology, which is a big reason why you need a monitoring system to help you see what's going on and what treatment works for you as an individual.

Natural Approaches to Common Chronic Conditions

Many physicians who use natural therapeutics have seen the reversal of common chronic conditions in their patients. It does take some work, and patience is required, often along with the guidance or supervision of an experienced health practitioner. There are many ways to approach these conditions, and I can recommend some good products with a history of success—but don't hesitate to seek help if you need it.

Sometimes you may only need to balance your terrain by using the monitoring system and making a few dietary adjustments, without using supplements—and that's always a good place to start. Balancing your pH is critical for your digestive tract's proper absorption of nutrients. Eliminate dairy products, coffee, alcohol, fried foods, and drugs if possible, or wean off of them as you start feeling better. Drink plenty of purified water.

A main goal in the natural therapeutic process is to improve digestion and eliminate intestinal and other inflammation. Many of the ingredients in Juice Plus+®, such as digestive enzymes, acidophilus, bacteria, and naturally occurring vitamin C, aid digestion and inflammation, which is another reason for including Juice Plus+® as a foundational food. (This is discussed further in Part Four of the book.)

A number of non-foundational supplements are useful for specific digestive issues. If you decide to try supplements, add one supplement to your program every three to five days and monitor its effect. If it causes more acidity, reduce the dose or discontinue the supplement and eat more alkaline foods. After a while, slowly increase your dose of the supplement. If it still produces an acidic reaction, it's time to try something else. (My book *Natural Healing with Herbs,* published by Hohm Press, describes herbal treatment suggestions.)

Consider the following non-foundational supplement options:

- Start taking digestive enzymes to aid your digestive process. Enzymes help decrease the bloating and fermentation that result from the buildup of undigested foods. (See the Enzymes chapter.)
- To repair and rebuild your gut lining, use supplemental glutamine, which is an amino acid found naturally in food. (See the Amino Acids chapter.) The cells that make up the lining of the intestinal tract use glutamine for energy and repair. Take 1,000–3,000 milligrams two or three times per day, between meals. (For more information, read Judy Shabert's book *The Ultimate Nutrient: Glutamine,* from Avery Publishing Group.)
- If your joints are affected (as in fibromyalgia), take proteolytic enzymes to reduce inflammation. These break down antibody-antigen complexes and reduce the buildup of fibrin formations that would otherwise impede much-needed blood flow to inflamed areas. Try a combination of bromelain and papain, or use a very effective enzyme formula called Wobenzym-n from Moss Nutrition (have your licensed healthcare practitioner call 800-851-5444).
- To restore your natural intestinal flora, use acidophilus and other probiotic or "friendly" bacteria (available in health food stores), taken between meals.
- To combat inflammation, use vitamin C (in ascorbate form, not ascorbic acid) at a dose of 3,000–5,000 milligrams daily. Make sure your vitamin C supplement also contains bioflavonoids. (See the Phytochemicals chapter.)
- The essential fatty acids EPA and DHA are excellent for joint and intestinal inflammation. Make sure they are combined with vitamin E, mixed tocopherols, and tocotrienols. You may need to purchase these supplements separately. (See the Fats chapter.)
- Sulfur is part of every cell's composition and is concentrated in the connective tissues and skin. Supplemental sulfur is great for sports

injuries and all inflammations of the joints and connective tissue. Use methylsulfonylmethane (MSM), a source of organic sulfur, at a daily dose of 1,000–10,000 milligrams taken with meals or with juice.

- Herbs that are used for inflammatory problems include boswellia, curcumin, white willow bark, guggul extract, and ginger root extract. Moss Nutrition combines these in a formula called Pain X. (See the chapter on Choosing the Right Diet and Supplements.)

While you experiment with the suggestions above, use the monitoring system to observe the effects of any supplements and dietary changes. Monitoring will tell you how you need to adjust your therapies to achieve balance. For instance, you might find that you need to eat more alkaline foods because of an acidic condition or detoxification; in such a case, you should use raw vegetable juices and green drinks and take your pH readings to see whether you need more buffering minerals (calcium, sodium, potassium, magnesium, and the like).

Remember, in some cases, you may get a little worse before you get better because the body is being burdened with the re-emergence of the toxins it's trying to eliminate from where they've been stored in the tissues. Keep your bowels moving; get colonics if necessary. To help eliminate toxins through the skin, sweat as much as possible and take Epsom salt baths or use a far-infrared sauna. (See the Environmental and Heavy Metal Toxicity chapter.)

If you have a Candida overgrowth problem or a fungal infection, do not simply try to "kill the bugs" with medication without balancing your terrain. At a pH in the body's normal range, yeast and fungus overgrowth will usually devolve back to their primitive form. Avoid all sugar products, coffee, dairy, and other acid-producing foods. A high-carbohydrate diet feeds yeast and fungus. Base your diet on lean organic meats and vegetables, especially low-starch vegetables and lots of raw salads. As a rule, limit grains; if you choose to eat them, make sure they are 100 percent whole grain or sprouted.

FREE RADICALS AND ANTIOXIDANTS

Parts of this chapter are a bit technical, but this is probably one of the most important chapters in the book. In the enormous amount of medical research conducted over the past thirty years, science has revealed a factor that is common to *every single degenerative disease.* It's not a virus or bacteria: it is cell damage due to free radicals.

You'll find it helpful to read the following definitions a few times before diving in:

Anti – against.

Pro – for.

Oxidize – to combine with oxygen.

Oxidant – a compound that oxidizes other compounds.

Oxidation – a chemical reaction in which electrons (one or more) are transferred from one atom or molecule to another.

Peroxidation – the production of unstable molecules containing more than the usual amounts of oxygen.

Antioxidant – a compound that prevents oxidation.

Free radical – an unstable and highly reactive atom or molecule that has one or more unpaired electrons in the outer shell; free radicals damage cells.

Oxidative stress – a condition in which the production of oxidants and free radicals exceeds the body's ability to defend itself.

Every normal molecule in your body has electrons spinning in pairs in its outer orbit. These paired electrons keep the molecule in perfect balance and acting in a very specific way according to its nature. If a molecule gains or loses one of these paired outer electrons for any reason, it becomes imbalanced and unstable—it is now a free radical. Unpaired electrons seek other electrons to pair with. Thus, free radicals are, in general, reactive, and they attack other molecules. That is one of the main ways that free radicals damage our tissues: by stealing electrons from the molecules in cell membranes, weakening the affected cells.

Free radicals can be found anywhere in the body. Where excess free radical activity destroys cells faster than the body can replace them, tissue death and even organ death occurs. Excess free radicals are the direct result of chemical exposure, emotional stress, physical exercise, sunlight, smoking, radiation, and drugs. And in addition to coming from these outside agents and special conditions, free radicals are generated by the body. The adult body at rest can produce 4 pounds of free radicals a year—and if it's exposed to smoke, other environmental toxins, and exercise, it can produce up to 20 pounds a year.

One type of free radical results from energy production by the mitochondria during normal cellular metabolism. I've mentioned mitochondria as the hundreds of "tiny furnaces" in each cell. Essentially, they combine oxygen with food—proteins, carbohydrates, and fats—to convert these nutrients into energy, in the form of ATP molecules. This oxidation process also releases free radicals. Some of the most common free radicals produced by your own body are superoxide, hydroxyl, and hydrogen peroxide, and these are responsible for considerable damage. On top of those, smoking, drugs, and other chemicals bring their own free radicals into your body, adding to what you've already produced.

The ultimate achievement for free radicals is to establish stability by either transferring their electrons to another atom or molecule or grabbing electrons from another atom or molecule. In either case, a free radical achieves stability only by creating another one, which then prowls the body, seeking another stable atom or molecule for electron transfer or stripping, and so on. This chain reaction can have disastrous consequences:

for instance, it's been calculated that a single free radical can damage about twenty-six molecules of polyunsaturated fat before losing its momentum. *(Pryor WA. Introduction to Free Radical Chemistry. Prentice-Hall, Englewood Cliffs, NJ, 1966.)* As you'll see later, the destruction of unsaturated fats is one of the most damaging effects of free radicals.

But don't despair, because your body has a natural defense against free radicals: antioxidants. The antioxidants you produce are the enzymes superoxide dismutase, catalase, and glutathione peroxidase. They neutralize free radicals, which can then be disposed of harmlessly. Your primary antioxidant source, however, is—or should be—your foods, particularly fruits and vegetables.

The Power of Fruits and Vegetables

Fruits and vegetables are rich in many helpful antioxidants. Antioxidants stop the free radical chain reaction by accepting renegade electrons into their own structure and hiding them away, rendering them harmless. It is clearly best for your health to counter free radicals with antioxidants, to prevent excessive free radical damage from pushing the body into a degenerative state that can create a focus of disease. If this disease process were to happen, part of your therapy would be to add more antioxidants to your diet. (See the Juice Plus+® chapter.)

Among the many antioxidants supplied by fruits and vegetables are vitamin E and the carotenoid beta-carotene, which defend cell membranes from free radical damage. Vitamin C protects the body's watery components. It seems especially adept at neutralizing free radicals from polluted air and cigarette smoke, and it can also restore oxidized vitamin E to its active state. Green leafy vegetables such as spinach and kale contain lutein, another powerful antioxidant.

Many minerals are antioxidants as well. Iodine, for example, has been shown to be an antioxidant on par with or better than vitamins C and E; its incorporation into cell membranes helps prevent lipid peroxidation. *(Smyth PP. Role of iodine in antioxidant defense in thyroid and breast disease. Biofactors 2003, 19:121-130; Tseng YL. Inhibition of lipid peroxidation. Lipids 1984, 19:96-102.)* The mineral selenium is a component of the antioxidant glutathione peroxidase, which protects red blood cells and cell membranes from free radicals, working in conjunction with vitamin E (or replacing it). Selenium-rich diets might reduce cancer risks.

We would all do well to follow the advice in Jean Carper's book *Stop Aging Now:* "Eat all the various fruits and vegetables you can. Nowhere will you find the anti-aging properties you get in fruits and vegetables. They possess countless known and unknown agents that transform your cells into fortresses against the free radical forces of aging. Much of what we call aging is really a fruit and vegetable deficiency." *(Carper J. Stop Aging Now. Harper-Collins Publishers, New York, NY, 1996.)*

Along those lines, a study reported in the *Journal of the American Medical Association* identified spinach as the food most apt to prevent cataracts in a group of elderly people. *(Seddon J, et al. Dietary carotenoids, vitamins A, C, and E, and advanced age-related macular degeneration. JAMA 1994 272:1413.)* Some reports suggest an inverse relationship between DNA damage and vegetable intake—that is, more vegetables, less damage. *(Djuric Z, et al. Oxidative DNA damage levels in blood from women at high risk for breast cancer are associated with dietary intakes of meats, vegetables, and fruits. J Am Diet Assoc 1998 98:524-528.)*

From an analysis of 4,500 scientific studies and papers on the relationship between cancer and diet, the American Institute for Cancer Research concluded that 40 percent of cancer cases worldwide could be prevented if people ate a low-fat, plant-based diet of fruits and vegetables. *(World Cancer Research Fund, American Institute for Cancer Research. Food, nutrition, and the prevention of cancer: a global perspective. American Institute for Cancer Research, Washington DC, 1997.)* Dr. Gladys Block, after reviewing 170 studies from different countries, stated similarly, "Eating fruits and vegetables regularly can slash your chances of getting cancer in half." *(Block G, et al. Fruit, vegetables, and cancer prevention: a review of the epidemiological evidence. Nutr Cancer 1992 18:1-29.)*

Epidemiological studies have also shown that people with high intakes of antioxidant-rich fruits and vegetables have lower rates of cancer. More specifically, vegetables in the cruciferous family—cabbage, kale, broccoli, cauliflower, and others—have been shown to contain phytochemicals (compounds found specifically in plants) that speed the removal of harmful estrogen from the body when it's fighting off breast cancer.

The research results in this area go on and on—and we have not yet even discovered all of the compounds in foods that can have anti-cancer and anti-aging effects. It seems too simple to be true, but when you realize that each fruit and vegetable contains hundreds or thousands of known and unknown phytochemicals, you can better understand the power of whole foods. It is always best to eat the whole food to get all of its synergistic phytochemicals and nutrients in nature's normal, optimal balance. (See the Phytochemicals chapter.)

Free Radicals and Aging

Fruit flies are a useful model for experiments related to aging because all of a fly's cells are the same chronological age, so the aging of the whole insect can be studied at once. Researchers have found that the aging of fruit fly cells is directly related to their ability to protect themselves from free radical damage. It has also been shown that for certain flies producing more antioxidants than others, their life spans are extended by one third.

Dr. Denham Harman identified a similar phenomenon in higher animals: "...the life span of mammals has a direct relationship to the amount of antioxidants found within their cells. For example, humans have longer life spans than other mammals because our cells contain more antioxidants than other mammals. Chimpanzees live longer than cats for the same reason. And then cats live longer than dogs, which live longer than mice, etc." (*Harman D. The aging process. Proc Natl Acad Sci 1981 78:7124-7128.*) Harman also describes research indicating that free radical damage could cause the formation of chemicals that, in turn, are responsible for the damage seen in the aging of cellular proteins, genetic material, and membranes. He concludes that dietary antioxidants including beta-carotene and vitamins C and E are essential nutrients in defense against free radicals.

It is clear that your ability to fight the ravages of aging from free radical damage depends on a combination of diet, lifestyle, genetics, and reducing your load of environmental toxins such as heavy metals and other chemicals. If you increase the antioxidants in your diet by eating plenty of fruit and vegetables, and if you also reduce your body's toxic load, you can defend yourself against free radical-induced oxidative stress, which at the cellular level is aging and disease.

Over time, if the body becomes inefficient in protecting itself from oxidative stress, its organs can begin to lose their functional abilities and degenerate. This is known as free radical pathology. If the affected organs are involved in digestion, digestive capabilities weaken. If the thyroid and adrenals are damaged by free radicals, the hormonal system gets depleted, and all sorts of problems can develop from reduced thyroid activity, insufficient adrenal output, and the like—basically, any disease or condition related to hormonal imbalance.

Many of the biomarkers or physical signs of aging are associated with oxidative stress. Although the effects of free radical damage can be seen throughout the body, they are especially evident in the organs with the highest oxygen levels, such as the heart, lungs, brain, and liver, as well as in the blood cells and skin. For instance, smoking causes excessive skin wrinkling because smoking produces free radicals that damage collagen and elastin, which are the proteins that hold the skin together. The same phenomenon occurs with sun-induced skin damage; ultraviolet rays penetrate the skin and induce the formation of free radicals that damage collagen in such a way that the affected skin puckers up in a fold.

Free Radicals, DNA, and Mitochondria

Not only do free radicals harm the outside of the cells that make up our organs and tissues, they can do damage inside our cells as well. Biochemist Bruce Ames says that from the oxygen we breathe, free radicals are produced that reach, and damage, the DNA of each cell in the body. Each cell can receive up to 10,000 free radical hits a day. Damaged DNA can cause cells to mutate into cancer cells—and DNA controls cell replication, which makes more. (*Ames BN. Endogenous oxidative DNA damage, aging, and cancer. Free Rad Res 1989 3:121-128.*)

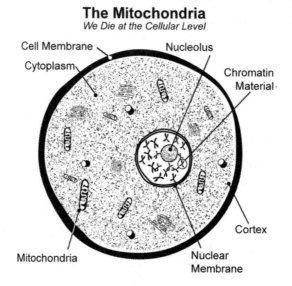

The Mitochondria
We Die at the Cellular Level

Cell Membrane

Cytoplasm

Nucleolus

Chromatin Material

Cortex

Mitochondria

Nuclear Membrane

Illustration by Eric Lindley

Studies have also shown that human aging may be related to free radical damage to the mitochondria. The DNA of the mitochondria is related to, but separate from, the DNA in the cell nucleus, and is much more vulnerable to damage. Ames recently found that mitochondrial DNA is about fifteen times more susceptible than nuclear DNA to oxidative stress from free radicals. If nuclear DNA is damaged, it may be repaired by an enzyme system within the cell, but no such enzyme system exists within the mitochondria, so their DNA mutations can pass to their "daughter" mitochondria. *(Richter C, et al. Normal oxidative damage to mitochondria and nuclear DNA is extensive. Nat Acad Sci 1988 85:6465-6467.)*

It's rather ironic that the processing of oxygen by mitochondria produces free radicals that can harm their own DNA if they're not protected by antioxidants such as vitamin E, co-enzyme Q-10, lipoic acid, glutathione, and superoxide dismutase. Fortunately, all of those protectors can be obtained through good nutrition. This is another example of how nutrients—or their lack—can affect gene expression, in this case determining your rate of aging at the cellular level. It's easy to see how molecules that affect you down to your DNA can be a major cause of disease. And as noted, free radicals are a factor in all chronic diseases.

Lipid Peroxidation

You've learned how your cells and even their DNA can be bombarded by free radicals up to 10,000 times a day. This is extremely problematic for the cell membrane's lipid layer, which is largely composed of fatty acids. Any time a fatty acid reacts with oxygen, it undergoes a process called lipid peroxidation, forming the free radical peroxide. (This is the same process that makes a fat or oil rancid.) Lipid peroxidation can damage and even destroy the cell's membrane and also the mitochondrial membranes.

As the membrane's lipids are turned rancid by free radicals, the membrane becomes rigid and hardens, and as a result, nutrients cannot get into the cell, or the cell is punctured and fluids escape. The damaged membrane loses its elasticity, its metabolic activities are hindered or lost completely, and the cell's health declines. It was formerly thought that cholesterol buildup caused this problem, but this is not the case.

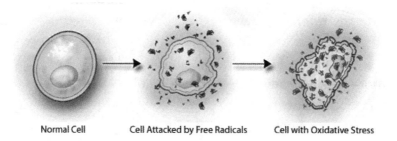

Normal Cell   Cell Attacked by Free Radicals   Cell with Oxidative Stress

Antioxidants come to the rescue by limiting cells' free radical exposure. Vitamin E, in particular, hangs out in the fatty layers of cells, where it neutralizes free radicals with help from an enzyme called lipid peroxidase. When enough antioxidants are available and in position, the cell membranes can retain their fluidity and function. But as the level of antioxidants in the body declines, aging and disease result. Is this is an inevitable process, or is it simply a correctible deficiency? I see it as the reason why at least one aspect of aging can be under your control. Taking in extra antioxidants—eating more fruits and vegetables—can help.

We've been told that cholesterol is the major culprit in cardiovascular disease, but this is far from the truth. (Refer to Uffe Ravnskov's book *The Cholesterol Myths,* from New Trends Publishing, for more information on false cholesterol propaganda.) Low-density lipoproteins (LDLs) and high-density lipoproteins (HDLs) are the other fats of interest in cardiovascular disease. LDL transfers cholesterol and triglycerides (another type of fats, from the diet and the liver) out of the bloodstream into the body's various tissues. HDL carries cholesterol from the arteries to the liver for breakdown and excretion.

The old thinking was that LDL is "bad" cholesterol, but it's just doing its natural job—the real problem is what happens to LDL when it's hit by free radicals. As free radicals attack the LDL and its "passenger" fats, the unsaturated fats in the triglycerides peroxidize. The resulting lipid peroxidation can overpower the available antioxidants. There is LDL in our arterial walls as well, and when it suffers free radical damage it is engulfed by our immune system's circulating scavenger cells, called macrophages. Unfortunately, in disposing of ruptured LDL, macrophages produce more free radicals.

Meanwhile, other circulating cells are attracted to the damage site and stick to the arterial wall, forming a plaque deposit. Over time, plaque buildup narrows coronary arteries, reducing blood flow to the heart. If a plaque accumulation bursts, blood clots can form and choke off the heart's blood supply, causing a heart attack. A similar blockage of blood supply to the brain can result in a stroke, loss of memory, dementia, and Alzheimer's disease.

In addition to LDLs, membranes also contain vitamin E and beta-carotene, which inhibit free radical damage from peroxidation. But if you smoke, are obese, or eat a high-fat diet, you need more antioxidants for protection. Although I do believe that supplemental antioxidants can be very helpful, it's always good to eat plenty of fruits and vegetables that naturally contain plant-derived antioxidants along with all the rest of their synergistic nutrients. Juice Plus+® can be beneficial in this regard. For example, researchers at the University of Maryland found that participants who consumed Juice Plus+® were better able to maintain elasticity of their arteries, even after a high-fat meal. (*Plotnick G. Effect of supplemental phytonutrients on impairment of the flow-mediated brachial artery vasoactivity after a single high-fat meal. J Am Coll Cardiol 2003 41:1744-1749.*)

Lipid peroxidation happens in places you might not expect. In the joints, a lubricant known as synovial fluid enables the bones to move without friction. Free radicals can oxidize the fat in synovial fluid so it loses its lubricating ability, and the joint becomes inflamed. An inflamed joint then produces more free radicals itself, and the ongoing chain reaction eventually causes arthritis.

Inflammation is a common effect of free radicals and can affect the stomach, intestinal tract, brain, and nervous system as well. Oxidant damage from free radical-induced lipid peroxidation is also a major cause of cataracts. Our eyes are constantly exposed to free radicals from ultraviolet radiation, chlorine, smoke, and pollution. The first layer to be attacked is the cornea, and the lens is particularly sensitive to free radical damage; vitamin E, however, has been known to stop this process.

Stop Free Radicals Before They Stop You

Free radical damage can occur anywhere in the body. And no matter what disease or condition you may have, free radicals are involved. The most logical thing to do is to beef up your antioxidant intake. Aging, cataracts, arthritis, Alzheimer's, cancer, autoimmune illnesses, hormone problems, the common cold, and fever—even depression, paranoia, anxiety, and panic attacks—are all associated with free radical damage or influenced by free radical activity. Oxidative stress is one of the major pathological processes in the body. There's that word again, "process." *Disease is a process.* If we understand that symptoms are a result of the process and are not the disease itself, we must go back to the beginning of the process to ask ourselves what started it, and what can we do to slow it down?

If you have any of the aforementioned conditions, taking supplemental antioxidants and eating more fruits and vegetables would definitely be a step in the right direction. You'll find plenty of antioxidant supplements at the health food store—it seems that scientists are finding out that almost every vitamin, mineral, and phytochemical so far identified has antioxidant qualities. Juice Plus+® is full of antioxidants! (See the Juice Plus+® chapter.)

Whether you're experiencing a chronic disease such as cancer, arthritis, lupus, or an inflammatory condition, or a more short-term condition such as a sports injury, cold, flu, allergy, canker sore, heartburn, or insomnia, monitoring your terrain can be a bottom-line therapy. Once any of these problems manifest, the pH and endocrine system have to be brought back into balance. The terrain must be normalized before total recovery is possible. Using the monitoring system will help you do that. With proper detoxification and supervision by a health-oriented physician, recovery is possible. Charting your blood pressure, temperature, and pH will bring what your body is experiencing more clearly into your awareness, so you can guide your body back into balance.

THE UNDIAGNOSED EPIDEMIC OF ENVIRONMENTAL AND HEAVY METAL TOXICITY

Now it's time to address the impact of external environmental toxins on your internal terrain, because our environment is becoming so toxic that we can't get away from its deadly poisons.

Our Toxic Environment

Perhaps you've heard of dioxins, which are chemical by-products from manufacturing plastics and pesticides and are a potent carcinogen (cause of cancer). Smoke-stacks pour dioxins and numerous other chemicals into the air; clouds carry the chemicals to every continent, poisoning the air, water, and soil; and the chemicals seep into plants, animals, and finally up the food chain to humans. Pesticides and herbicides are sprayed on our lawns, crops, and weeds; animals are sprayed when crops are aerially sprayed. Before food goes to market, it's sprayed again with fungicides. Our schools, businesses, churches, restaurants, and golf courses are also sprayed with pesticides. Plastic wraps give off chemicals called phthalates, which leach into our foods and then attach themselves to our cells, leading to hormone imbalance, disrupted brain chemistry, and even cancer. Some of these chemicals take thirty years to dissolve even half-way. They never go away; we're continually bombarded by them.

All of these chemicals also end up in mothers' breast milk and are transferred to our children. Some studies have found breast milk to contain as much as eighteen times the normal amount of dioxin. No wonder cancer in children has increased in the last twenty years. Studies have even shown that the breast milk of Inuit Indian mothers contains very high levels of modern chemical poisons. *(Johansen BE. The Inuit's struggle with dioxins and other organic pollutants. Am Ind Quart 2002 26:479-*

490.) Who would have imagined that Eskimos living in the pristine Arctic could experience such environmental toxicity?

We're told that small amounts of these poisons are harmless—this may or may not be true. But what we aren't told is that the body has no way of getting rid of some of these chemicals, so they're stockpiled in our tissues over the years, causing what we've come to call aging. We then suffer from what might have been avoidable conditions: high blood pressure, prostate and thyroid cancers, multiple sclerosis (MS), osteoporosis, joint degeneration, heart failure, and autoimmune diseases such as lupus and rheumatoid arthritis.

Studies conducted by the U.S. Environmental Protection Agency (EPA) have revealed that 100 percent of Americans harbor some environmental toxins in their fatty tissue. *(U.S. Environmental Protection Agency. Chlorinated dioxins and furans in the general U.S. population: NHATS FY87 results. EPA-560/5-91-003. Office of Toxic Substances, Washington DC, 1991.)* Although the problem is inescapable and a tremendous health hazard, it is not even considered by most primary care physicians. But the day will come when public awareness will demand a change.

Toxins in the Home Environment

Years ago, insulating homes and offices with a foam formaldehyde material was very popular. Foam formaldehyde is also found in sofas and mattresses. Seemingly out of nowhere, people began developing symptoms such as depression, arthritis, asthma, nausea, and migraine headaches. Some people were totally incapacitated, and some took years to recover—because the issue of environmental sensitivities was not yet understood, and because people didn't realize that many seemingly harmless materials were out-gassing (slowly giving off) toxins.

Carpets out-gas more than a dozen different chemicals that can cause illness: benzene, toluene, butadiene, styrene, and methacrylates, to name a few. Experiments have shown that putting a patch of carpet in a cage of mice caused all the mice to die by the next morning. Other toxins come from paints, solvents, grease, gas dryers, washing machines, and the various chemicals stored in our garages and basements. Faulty furnaces release poisons causing stomach problems, depression, and lung infection. Construction materials such as plasticizers, wallpaper, and the pressed wood used in cabinets and drawers also release poisons into the air.

Large amounts of these out-gassed poisons enter your body through your pores. The smaller the body is, the more concentrated the poison accumulation will be; this means that children are particularly susceptible to its effects. Some people are also more sensitive than others because they are already carrying a load of other poisons in their tissues. Even our pets are affected by the chemicals in our homes. Everyone should have air purifiers in their most comfortable rooms to prevent toxic air syndrome.

Meanwhile, molds that can develop from leaky roofs and cellars, humidifiers, and air-conditioners are very toxic to your body as well. As described previously in this book, molds produce mycotoxins that can even be cancer-causing in certain situations, depending on the individual's pre-existing toxic load and other biochemical factors.

Hundreds of different chemicals are present in our water. You absorb them when you bathe and through cooking and drinking. Water is poisoned by industrial wastes and agricultural runoffs of chemical fertilizers, heavy metals, and pesticides. The fluoride put into drinking water and toothpaste damages digestive enzymes and accumulates in arteries and joints, causing calcification and joint damage. Fluoride has been linked to osteoporosis and certain forms of cancer. Accumulated fluoride can cause learning difficulties, birth defects, and flu symptoms. Beware of fluoride added to infant formulas, foods, juices, and tooth treatments—even Prozac. Meanwhile, a national survey of 39,000 children showed no significant difference in tooth decay between children drinking fluoridated versus non-fluoridated water. *(Yiamouyiannis J. Water fluoridation and tooth decay: results from the 1986-1987 national survey of U.S. school children. Fluoride 1990 23:55-67.)*

Chloride is added to water to kill bacteria and other organisms. In addition to drinking it, you absorb chloride through your pores. Unfortunately, it can raise your cholesterol levels and damage your blood vessel walls. Around every cell in the body is a membrane with a lipid (fatty) layer. When lipid peroxidation by chloride damages this layer, the membrane leaks, inhibiting the cell's metabolism and possibly causing its death.

One way to minimize water toxicity is to have a filter installed at water's first point of entry into your home, so you will no longer be showering, bathing, and brushing your teeth with poisoned water. The next thing to improve is your everyday cooking and drinking water. Drinking alkaline water helps prevent the host of negative health effects of over-acidification. High Tech Health (800-794-5355) offers a good alkaline water machine; tell them you read about their product in this book and ask for information on all their products. I have had success with their alkaline machine and far-infrared sauna. There are also many other options on the market.

Toxins and the Disease Process

Columbia University released a public health report stating that 95 percent of all cancer is caused by diet and environment. So which of the two is more to blame? It's a moot point, because the poisons in our environment and in our foods are the same. What's the difference if a pesticide directly sprayed on crops makes us sick or if it seeps into the soil and poisons our food supply that way?

In the book *Detoxify or Die*, which everybody should read, Dr. Sherry Rogers tells a chilling true story about a group of children who jumped and played in the spray from a spray-truck that came down the street. As it turned out, they were playing in DDT, which has an incubation period in the body of twenty to forty years. In adulthood, these folks developed baffling illnesses: MS, Parkinson's disease, fibromyalgia, fatigue, and cancer. *(Rogers SA. Detoxify or Die. Sand Key Company, Sarasota, FL, 2003.)* This story also demonstrates "different strokes for different folks," as a toxin can cause a number of different conditions depending on the genetic make-up of the affected individuals.

Any one of the toxins I've described—and there are many, many more—can cause a focus of disease in the body. But when you've gone to your doctor with a health problem, have you ever been asked whether you'd been exposed to any environmental poisons? Have you ever been tested for environmental poisons that could be related to your condition? Most doctors never do this type of work—and yet, these poisons are directly related to our modern-day epidemics.

Toxins are tissue-selective, meaning that they settle in certain areas in the body. Phthalates, for example, are endocrine gland disruptors because of their affinity for hormone-producing tissues. They mimic hormones, block hormone production, and create chemical imbalances, leading to fatigue, mood swings, memory loss, depression, and loss of libido. They can also cause cancer in breasts, prostate, and testicles. Recall the disease process: chemicals such as phthalates can be the cause, producing a focus; then, as a symptom of toxin accumulation, cancer results, and it spreads to produce numerous symptoms far distant from the original cause. Treating symptoms without eliminating the cause (in this case, toxic buildup) is like a cat chasing its tail.

Once these poisons have gotten in, we do not possess sufficient detoxification mechanisms to eliminate them completely. We have to rely on procedures such as chelation and sweating therapies to aid the body in eliminating them, as described later in this chapter.

Heavy Metal Toxicity

Heavy metal toxicity is a worldwide epidemic. These metals are the oldest toxins known to mankind, and the list of illnesses they cause is enormous: MS, autism, allergies, gut problems, dementia, Alzheimer's disease, anxiety, depression, cancer, fibromyalgia, fatigue, blurred vision, dental problems (from amalgam fillings and root canals), heart disease, chemical sensitivity, leukemia, autoimmune disease, and schizophrenia—and that's only a partial list.

Accumulated heavy metals in the body cause an ongoing acidifying reaction, promoting the development of yeast and fungus. Heavy metals also destroy enzymes in the digestive tract, causing food to ferment, which releases more acids, which are then absorbed into the bloodstream and lymphatic system—and the causal chain continues.

Heavy metals destroy fatty acids as well, thereby cutting down cellular uptake of nutrients and oxygen; this causes the tissues to give up alkaline minerals, producing mineral deficiencies. Furthermore, heavy metals displace needed minerals such as zinc, copper, iron, manganese, and magnesium. Think of all the problems that can come of being deficient in just one of these minerals—zinc, for instance, is involved in over 100 enzyme functions in the body. And if you are deficient in zinc, you absorb more of the heavy metal cadmium.

Heavy metals are in foods, soil, cigarette smoke, cookware, and more. As they accumulate in our bodies for ten to twenty years, they start to cause immune system damage, panic attacks, depression, and kidney damage. They lodge in certain organs, joints, and bones depending on your individual constitution, genetic make-up, and biochemistry. Chronic fatigue is one of the first symptoms you'll notice. This occurs because the metals disturb the mitochondria, which are the energy-synthesis centers within your cells.

Because heavy metals accumulate in the body over a period of years and symptoms of their toxicity come on slowly, they aren't often thought of as a cause of chronic disease. But you now know that disease is a process, and that if you change the process, you'll change the disease. By monitoring your terrain and making adjustments with the proper nutrition, supplements, fatty acids, enzymes, and minerals, you can halt this process in its tracks. If you find your terrain difficult to balance, you should get a blood or urine test specifically for heavy metals.

I'll describe arsenic, aluminum, cadmium, lead, and mercury in detail. There are others such as platinum, tungsten, copper, nickel, and beryllium. But after reading about a few, you'll begin to see what a serious problem any heavy metal can be.

A note to prospective parents: please get checked for heavy metal toxicity before you conceive. These metals cross the placental barrier to the fetus and are deposited in the developing brain tissue and other organs. Children born with heavy metal toxicity can experience any of the serious symptoms and conditions detailed below.

Arsenic. Arsenic overload can cause dermatitis, cardiac disease, respiratory infection, peripheral neuropathy, liver disease, chronic fatigue, and Reynard's symptoms. It can even stop your bone marrow from making blood cells. Arsenic is found in pesticides, herbicides, fungicides, wood preservatives, tobacco, paint, seafood, meat, fish, and poultry.

Aluminum. This metal permeates our air, water, soil, and food. The average person consumes 3–10 milligrams of aluminum daily. Aluminum is used in cookware, cooking utensils, and foil. Excessive use of antacids is a common cause of aluminum toxicity. Mylanta, Maalox, Asphodel, and other drugs have a high aluminum hydroxide content, as do over-the-counter anti-inflammatory drugs and pain remedies such as arthritis pain formulas, Bufferin, and Vanquish. Several douche preparations including Massengill and Summer's Eve contain aluminum. It is also found in baking powder, antiperspirants, deodorants, beer (from the cans), bleached flours, and parmesan and grated cheeses.

Many symptoms of aluminum toxicity are similar to those of Alzheimer's disease; others include osteoporosis, colic, gastrointestinal disturbance, memory loss, softening of the bones, and weak and aching muscles. Aluminum compounds can accumulate in the brain, disturbing nerve impulses, causing seizures, and reducing mental faculties. Post-mortem examination of Alzheimer's victims has revealed four times the normal amount of aluminum in their brains' nerve cells.

Cadmium. Cadmium toxicity can cause emphysema, chronic fatigue, protein-losing kidney disease, liver and prostate cancers, hypertension, angina, hormone imbalance, hypothyroidism, depression, and high cholesterol levels. Cadmium is unavoidable. It is found in cigarettes, commercial foods, nickel-cadmium batteries, and shellfish and other seafood, and is emitted in vehicle exhaust and the burning of fossil fuels. Chemically treated water often contains cadmium. The scary part is that it takes the body ten to twenty years to get rid of just half of its accumulated cadmium without assistance.

Lead. This metal can be found in large amounts in food, water, and the air, especially in areas where a lot of motor traffic produces a lot of exhaust, sending lead through the air directly into our lungs. Lead-based paints used in older homes put children at risk from flaking paint chips with high lead content. Because lead is chemically similar to calcium, it is handled by the body as if it were calcium and is initially distributed to the blood and soft membranes; it can also be distributed to bones and teeth.

Acute lead poisoning causes convulsions, but with a gradual buildup of lead, there is no sudden onset of symptoms. Initial long-term symptoms include vertigo, clumsiness, anorexia, abdominal pains, vomiting, irritability, and insomnia. As lead levels rise, convulsions, delirium, and anxiety may occur. Because lead reacts with calcium and is secreted in saliva, it will eventually show up as a purplish or black deposit, called "lead lines," at the gum line in the mouth.

Mercury. Mercury is probably the worst metal offender. It is found in shellfish, large fish, paints, tattoo inks, ceramics, exhaust fumes, immunizations, and dental fillings. Mercury toxicity has been linked to autoimmune disease, heart disease, infection, depression, schizophrenia, autism, MS, and leukemia.

In the past decade, the public has become aware of mercury exposure from silver dental fillings. Silver-mercury amalgams (mixtures) have been used to fill cavities for more than 180 years. These fillings contain 50 percent mercury by weight, which vaporizes from them continuously; its release is intensified by chewing, brushing, and hot liquids. The vaporized mercury is then absorbed through the digestive tract. A person with a mere eight fillings has a daily 10-microgram mercury exposure.

Research on sheep and monkeys has demonstrated that dental mercury accumulates in all tissues and is highest in the kidney and liver. Human autopsies have shown that the brain and kidney tissues of people with mercury fillings contain significantly higher amounts of mercury than people without those fillings. A comparison of brain tissue from Alzheimer's victims versus an age-matched group of non-Alzheimer's subjects also found a significantly higher amount of mercury in the Alzheimer's group.

Mercury from the mouth can form the compound methyl mercury, which passes readily through all membranes and other physiological barriers and can end up anywhere in the body. Guess where it likes to deposit itself? The brain. Mercury can also travel directly from the teeth to the brain in its original form. I have known several dentists, exposed to high levels of mercury over the years, who suffered from depression, fatigue, and anxiety, and ultimately had to quit their dental practices because of severe emotional problems—all linked to mercury toxicity.

If you decide to get your amalgam fillings removed, make sure you choose a "biological dentist" who has experience in removing them. He or she should prepare you by suggesting a natural chelating substance to be used before and after filling removal, to bind with mercury and escort it out of your body. *Chelation Therapy*

My mercury toxicity experience. I went through a year of symptoms including chronic fatigue, anxiety, and sleeplessness. Every traditional test was done on me, only to find absolutely nothing wrong. Finally, I was introduced to Dr. Charles Gant—and thank goodness for Dr. Gant. He immediately asked if I had been checked for heavy metals; he had the blood test done and found that I was loaded with mercury. I went through detoxification; it took two years before I was normal. I couldn't work or exercise, and I stayed in my bedroom for nine months.

My daughter brought food to my room, but I'd eat very little. This taught me, by the way, why it was so hard to get my clients to eat healthy: while I was this sick and my chemistry was so far out of balance, the only food I craved was junk food, especially potato chips. As my chemistry changed, so did my craving, until I was back to normal. It took two years because for the first nine months I was trying to do it myself, taking every supplement under the sun. I thought I was doing the right thing, but when you're toxic, your liver is already working overtime and can't process such large amounts of nutrients. Another lesson learned: too much of a good thing can be a bad thing.

In *Detoxify or Die*, Dr. Rogers notes that accumulated mercury can cause peripheral neuropathy, chronic fatigue, and fibromyalgia. These symptoms can also present themselves during the detoxification process. When I was going through mercury detox, my body sometimes felt like it was on fire, especially my back and chest. But all of the discomfort passed once I was detoxified properly.

Heavy Metal Detoxification Products

There are several tests to detect heavy metal toxicity and several ways to eliminate metals from your body. Tests are offered by Metametrix (800-221-4640) and Doctor's Data (800-323-2784); your licensed healthcare practitioner can order them. If your doctor won't help you with testing or treatment for a suspected metal problem, find another doctor. Specialists called environmental doctors know how to work with problems caused by metal overload. You may have to travel to find one, but we're talking about your health, and your health is your primary responsibility.

Dr. Joseph Mercola maintains an informative Web site, www.mercola.com, which may help you locate a physician experienced in detoxification methods. You can also contact the American Academy of Environmental Medicine: 6505 East Central Avenue, #296, Wichita, KS 67206; phone 316-684-5500, fax 316-684-5709; www.aaemonline.org.

If you do have a metal problem, please do not try to detoxify yourself. Specific remedies must be used, and the process of elimination has to be monitored to prevent kidney damage or other problems while the body is ridding itself of the toxins. You should only undergo detoxification for accumulated heavy metals slowly and safely, with professional guidance and supervision.

Chelation therapy. Taken from the Greek word meaning "claw," the term "chelation" refers to the binding of metal molecules by certain compounds. Chelation therapy uses a chelating agent to carry metals out of the body. Some chelating agents can be administered intravenously, such as the laboratory-synthesized protein called ethylene diamine tetraacetic acid (EDTA). EDTA eliminates heavy metals and is also used to unclog arteries in cardiovascular disease; in many cases, bypass surgery may be avoided when such a therapy is used. I have personally taken an oral chelating agent called Metal-Free®, available from Body Health (877-804-3258).

Metal-Free® is derived from naturally occurring substances by a process of microfermentation. Its active ingredients are peptides that have a very high affinity for heavy metals and bind with them so they can be more readily excreted from the body. Research on Metal-Free® has been done in lab cultures, mice and rats, and humans. Human testing showed 100–700 percent increases in heavy metal excretion compared to normal excretion. Adding Metal-Free® to a mercury detox protocol, for example, speeds the process by 30–50 percent. It has been used in thousands of clinics for more than eight years and has an excellent safety record.

Chelation therapy is someone everyone should become familiar with. (The Web has plenty of information on the subject, and you can read the following books: *Chelation Therapy* by Morton Walker and Hitendra Shah, published by McGraw-Hill, and *Forty-Something Forever* by Harold and Arline Brecher, from Health Savers Press.)

Sweating Therapy for Toxin Elimination

What is the best way to get rid of pesticides, heavy metals, hydrocarbons, dioxin, and most of the other chemical toxins in your body? Use a far-infrared sauna. Usually I don't suggest something so expensive ($2,000–$3,000), but when you consider that 70,000 chemicals have been introduced into our environment, that's 70,000 reasons I believe we should all have a sauna in our homes.

You have read in this chapter about the prevalence of toxic chemicals in the air, water, and food supply, about their buildup and migration to specific sites, and about their eventual symptoms, damage to vital organs, and blockage of neurological pathways. But instead of approaching this problem by detoxifying the body, conventional medicine prescribes drugs that only make matters worse by poisoning the body further: HNG-COA inhibitors (for high cholesterol), MAOIs and SSRIs (for depression), H_2 blockers (for heartburn), alpha- and beta-blockers (for heart problems and blood pressure), and acetyl cholinesterase inhibitors (for Alzheimer's).

This form of treatment adds another chemical to the accumulated toxins that are interfering with the body's natural biochemical processes. The body is already working hard to get rid of these poisons through its built-in chemical and metabolic pathways to final elimination in sweat, stool, and urine. So the last thing you want to do is shut down any of these pathways with an inhibiting or blocking drug.

Technology has now brought us the far-infrared sauna, which has proven to be one of the best and safest ways to rid the body of toxicity of all kinds, including accumulated heavy metals and chemicals. As you may know, energy exists in a spectrum of various wavelengths. At the short end of the spectrum are gamma rays, then x-rays, and then ultraviolet; next comes the range of visible light; and at the long end of the spectrum is the healing infrared range. The rays used in the far-infrared sauna are some of the longest wavelengths, 4–20 microns, which also happen to be the rays used by plants in photosynthesis. Your body radiates infrared energy, and you can absorb 93 percent of the infrared rays you're exposed to. In the sauna, the rays penetrate the body to a depth of 1.5 inches on all sides and cause it to sweat out toxins. (Everybody should read *Sauna Therapy* by Dr. Lawrence Wilson; see www.drlwilson.com.)

Plenty of research has demonstrated how sweating eliminates these poisons. Dr. William Rea, Medical Director of the Environmental Health Center in Dallas, Texas, has sweated thousands of patients in far-infrared saunas to improve their health. In one of Dr. Rea's studies, 210 patients with a variety of symptoms received one or two forty-minute sauna sessions daily for thirty days, and even within this short period, 63 percent showed decreased levels of toxic chemicals. *(Rea WJ, et al. Reduction of chemical sensitivity by means of heat depuration, physical therapy and nutritional supplementation in a controlled environment. J Nutr Environ Med 1996 6:141-148.)*

But not just any sauna will do; it has to be far-infrared to produce the greatest detoxifying effect. In addition, this sauna has been proven to reduce lactic acid buildup, stimulate endorphins, kill bacteria and parasites, improve blood flow to the heart, and stop swelling. It has even been shown to be beneficial for cardiovascular disease and is one of the safest ways to induce sweating for heat-sensitive cardiac patients. For more information on far-infrared saunas and sweating therapy, contact High Tech in Boulder, Colorado (800-794-5355).

The far-infrared sauna is tolerable by patients with all types of chronic disease. But, of course, you must be careful—start slowly, and don't overdo it. Specific instructions for use come with the sauna package. If you begin to feel sick, nauseous, panicky, or faint, get out. As your toxic load begins to diminish, you'll be able to stay in for longer periods; usually thirty to sixty minutes is plenty. You may be able to find some doctors in your area who use the far-infrared sauna. I think everybody should have one, as we're constantly exposed to toxic chemicals.

You will be sweating out minerals, vitamin C, and water, so you should always take vitamin C, calcium, magnesium, and other minerals before and after your sauna session. Drink alkaline water while you're in the sauna and for the next hour afterward. You'll feel wonderful again. A good source for minerals is Reality Health Research (877-454-3313). Their mineral supplements are in elemental form and easy to absorb. Happy sweating!

DISEASE-FIGHTING PHYTOCHEMICALS

Whole foods supply a cornucopia of beneficial compounds in a synergistic balance that can never be duplicated by man. Raw foods that are not processed or cooked have a God-given balance that co-exists as interconnected food elements: vitamins, minerals, enzymes, proteins, carbohydrates, and fats. Along with these traditional nutrients is another huge group of naturally occurring chemicals that are now known to benefit the body as well—you'll recognize their name as the current nutritional buzz-word "phytochemicals." The term is derived from the prefix "phyto," which means plant. Phytochemicals, also called phytonutrients, are compounds found naturally in fruits, vegetables, seeds, nuts, and legumes. There are literally hundreds and maybe even thousands of phytochemicals in each species of plant.

Phytochemicals naturally protect their plant against viruses, bacteria, and fungus. There has been a lot of interest in these compounds because many of them act as free radical scavengers in and around our cells; slow the aging process; support and strengthen the immune system; and even reduce the risk of cancer, heart disease, and inflammatory conditions. Researchers have identified various specific phytochemicals as anti-aging and anti-cancer agents because they have been shown to modify gene expression. As you have read in previous chapters, our genes don't change, but their activity and effects can be modified by the foods we eat.

Foods can be seen as having many levels of expression themselves. Not only do they contain all the familiar vitamins and minerals, but as we look deeper into the healing properties of herbs, fruits, and vegetables, we find hundreds of phytochemicals energetically combined and working with these known nutrients. We have also realized that cooking and processing our foods destroys many of these beneficial substances. Although some phytochemicals do remain in cooked foods, the only way to get them in their entirety and in their most useful forms is to eat raw or slightly steamed vegetables and fruits, or to drink fresh vegetable and fresh fruit juices. And because we know that many different phytochemicals in fruits and vegetables have only recently been identified, we must deduce that there could still be as many or more unknown substances yet to be discovered in these foods.

An important consideration is how all of the nutritive substances work together to protect plants from dangers in their environment. It's logical to conclude that if you removed 100 of a plant's naturally protective chemicals, it would probably die or at least be altered in some significant way, just as we've all seen plants die or have leaves turn brown in deficient soil. The optimal function of any one of these chemicals depends on the presence of the rest of the chemicals normally found along with it— if you remove even one substance from the mix, you don't get the same expression or functional result.

Isolated Nutrients versus Whole Foods

We know we need our vitamins and minerals, but we know at times they just don't seem to work. As with phytochemicals, once you remove vitamins or minerals from their source, from their context of nutritional companions, you may get a completely different activity.

An analogy: if you're listening to a symphony performed by eighty musicians and you remove one violin, not only is there something missing in the symphony, but the singled-out violin has lost its synergistic companions and, consequently, some of its own identity. It may be able to function at some level alone, but its solo performance will never be what it can achieve within the whole orchestra. The same idea applies to taking individual nutrients and thinking they'll act in the same way that they would if you'd eaten them in a whole food. We need both—individual supplements and whole foods—but they are not alike.

As mentioned, many unknown components contribute to the constitution of our foods and affect the performance of the nutrients that we do know about. When clients ask why they should make the effort to eat whole foods when they're taking a multivitamin supplement, I have a two-part answer. First, no scientist could possibly produce a pill in which thousands of substances work together as they do in a plant produced by nature; second, a supplement manufacturer obviously can't produce phytochemicals that haven't been discovered yet. So even if you use a multivitamin, you should still eat foods as close to nature as possible.

Eat More Fruits and Vegetables

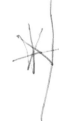

In general, it has been found that people who eat higher amounts of fruits and vegetables have about half the risk of developing cancer. *(Block G, et al. Fruit, vegetables and cancer prevention: a review of the epidemiological evidence. Nutr Cancer 1992 18:1-29.)* Studies show, for instance, that people who eat fruits and vegetables are less likely to develop cancers that involve epithelial cells in organs such as the lungs, cervix, esophagus, stomach, colon, and pancreas. *(Steinmetz KA, Potter JD. Vegetables, fruit, and cancer, II. Mechanisms. Cancer Causes Control 1991 2:427-442.)* These whole foods have also been shown to contain substances that are precursors used by the body to build hormones.

And yet, a recent survey of eating habits revealed that only one in eleven Americans meets the guideline of three vegetable servings and two fruit servings daily. *(Subar AS, et al. 5 A Day for Better Health: a baseline study of Americans' fruit and vegetable consumption. National Cancer Institute, NIH, Rockville, MD, 1991.)* Furthermore, nutrient-dense vegetables such as kale, beets, and parsley weren't even mentioned by that survey's respondents;

most Americans don't eat those very often, and consider iceberg lettuce and celery to be rich in nutrients. From more than twenty years of practicing holistic therapies, I can say that a lack of high-quality, nutrient-dense food, and the deficiencies that result from this lack, are major factors in the cause of disease and should be considered by physicians in their treatment of ill patients.

A Primer on Phytochemicals

A number of phytochemicals assist the body in its own detoxification processes. Glutathione S-transferase (GST), for example, is a very important enzyme used by the body to detoxify cancer-producing chemicals. Phytochemicals that stimulate GST activity are considered cancer inhibitors: among them are the dithiolthiones and isothiocyanates found in broccoli, cabbage, and other cruciferous vegetables; the phthalides in celery seeds; the liminoids in citrus; and the curcumins in ginger and turmeric, to name just a few. A study in the Netherlands reported that people who ate Brussels sprouts had more GST than people who did not eat Brussels sprouts. (*Zheng G-Q, et al. Stimulation of glutathione S-transferase and inhibition of carcinogenesis in mice by celery seed oil constituents. In: Food Phytochemicals for Cancer Prevention I. Fruits and Vegetables. MJ Huang, et al. (eds). ACS, Washington DC, 1994; Lam LKT, et al. Inhibition of chemically induced carcinogenesis by citrus liminoids. In: Food Phytochemicals for Cancer Prevention I. Fruits and Vegetables. M-J Huang, et al. (eds). American Chemical Society, Washington DC, 1994; Bland JS, Benum SH. Genetic Nutritioneering. Keats Publishing, New Canaan, CT, 1999.*)

Let me introduce you to several significant groups of phytochemicals and some particularly powerful foods:

Phenols. Phenols protect plants from oxidative stress and perform the same function in humans. Phenols also help block specific enzymes that cause inflammation.

Flavonoids. This is a group of more than 1,500 phenols that enhance the effects of vitamin C. Hesperidin and quercetin are examples. Flavonoids are mainly anti-inflammatory, but also act as free radical scavengers and protect against platelet aggregation, allergic reactions, and liver toxins. Among other benefits, taking vitamin C with flavonoids helps strengthen tiny capillaries.

Quercetin. This specific flavonoid appears to protect against heart disease by inhibiting platelet aggregation, thereby reducing the risk of blood clots. Quercetin is also used to reduce inflammation in sports injuries and to reduce the problematic release of histamine from mast cells during asthma, bronchitis, and allergic reactions.

Glucosinolates. Found in cruciferous vegetables, glucosinolates activate liver detoxification and help block enzymes that promote cancer growth. Glucosinolates also help regulate the activity of cytokines, which are hormone-like substances that help coordinate immune system responses and control inflammation.

Phytosterols. These lipid (fat) compounds are similar to cholesterol. Some phytosterols are found in vegetables but are most concentrated in seeds. Phytosterols from seeds block the development of breast, colon, and prostate diseases, reduce inflammation, and help eliminate excess cholesterol from the body.

Carotenoids. Carotenoids are a group of approximately 450 pigments found in yellow, orange, red, and green fruits and vegetables, berries of all types, grapes, and black currants. They stimulate the immune system and reduce the risk of heart disease and cancer. You've probably heard of the carotenoid beta-carotene. *(Ziegler RG. Vegetables, fruits, and carotenoids and the risk of cancer. Am J Clin Nutr 1991 53 (suppl):251S-259S; van Poppel G, Goldbohm RA. Epidemiologic evidence for beta-carotene and cancer prevention. Am J Clin Nutr 1995 62:13938S-14002S.)*

Lycopene. Lycopene is the reddish pigment in tomatoes. In the body, it is deposited in certain tissues such as the prostate gland (an example of selective nutrition). Lycopene helps prevent prostate cancer and heart disease.

Lutein. Lutein is an antioxidant in the carotenoid family. It is found in green leafy vegetables such as spinach, kale, leeks, and romaine lettuce. Lutein protects against age-related macular degeneration, a leading cause of blindness in people older than sixty-five.

Zeaxanthin. This phytochemical is also found in large amounts in spinach. Both zeaxanthin and lutein (above) have been found to protect the eyes against degenerative conditions.

Ellagic acid. Ellagic acid acts as a natural pesticide in strawberries and raspberries. It also helps fight against cancers in humans.

Indoles. Indoles are potent cancer-fighters found in broccoli, cabbage, kale, and Brussels sprouts.

Sulforaphane. This compound has been shown to help prevent colon cancer. Sulforaphane is found in cruciferous vegetables such as broccoli, cauliflower, kale, Brussels sprouts, cabbage, collard greens, and turnips.

Anthocyanidins. These water-soluble flavonoids (above) strengthen the collagen protein in soft tissues, tendons, ligaments, and bones, and are therefore particularly useful for athletes. Anthocyanidins also neutralize free radicals that damage soft tissue. More than 125 anthocyanidins of interest have been found so far.

Catechins. Catechins are a group of well-known antioxidant flavonoids found in green tea.

Citrus fruits. Citrus fruits contain numerous phytochemicals with a wide range of activities including anti-tumor and antioxidant properties and activation of the detoxifying P-450 enzyme system. *(Attaway JA. Citrus juice flavonoids with anti-carcinogenic and anti-tumor properties. In: Food Phytochemicals for Cancer Prevention I. Fruits and Vegetables. M-J Huang, et al. (eds). American Chemical Society, Washington DC, 1994.)* An orange contains more than 170 known phytochemicals. *(Pierson HF. Over 170 phytonutrients in an orange. Oral presentation at 77th Annual Meeting of the American Dietetic Association, Orlando, FL, 1994.)* Grapefruit and oranges contain nomilin and limonin, which activate the enzyme GST to help neutralize toxic substances in the body. Citrus pulp is rich in glucarate, which helps prevent breast cancer.

Flaxseed. Flaxseed has been shown to lower cholesterol and is a good source of omega-3 fats. *(Cunnane SC, et al. High alpha-linolenic acid (Linum usitalissimum): some nutritional properties in humans. Br J Nutr 1993 69:443.)* Flaxseed contains plant lignans, which appear to be anti-carcinogenic. In the colon, lignans are converted into phyto-estrogens, which are similar in structure to estrogen and can inhibit the growth of estrogen-stimulated breast cancers. *(Hirano T, et al. Antiproliferative activity of mammalian lignan derivatives against the human breast carcinoma cell line, ZR-75-1. Cancer Invest 1990 8:595-602; Serraino M, Thompson LU. The effect of flaxseed supplementation* *on the initiation and promotional stages of mammary tumorigenesis. Nutr Cancer 1992 17:153-159.)*

Red wine and grape juice. These contain phenols and red anthocyanins, which are antioxidants that protect against lipid oxidation, thereby protecting against heart disease. *(Frankel EN, et al. Inhibition of oxidation of human low-density lipoprotein by phenolic substances in red wine. Lancet 1993 341:454-457.)*

Garlic and onions. Garlic and onions are rich in allyl sulfides, which tend to reduce cancer risk, lower total cholesterol, and help reduce blood clotting.

Phytochemicals and Your Terrain

The primer above is just a taste—much more information is available. My point is to emphasize the wealth of known and unknown phytochemicals that exist in fruits, vegetables, seeds, nuts, and legumes. (I'm not including grains in this discussion, because not everyone should be eating grains.) You can surely see how important it is to eat whole foods. Vitamin and mineral supplements definitely play helpful roles in balancing your terrain, maintaining your health, and dealing with illness—but whole, raw, unprocessed food is vital.

All of the nutrients your body needs must be readily available for your cellular functions of building, repairing, and growing to occur as they should. The principle of selective nutrition holds that at any second, any one of your trillions of cells may require a specific phytochemical, vitamin, mineral, or enzyme. If that substance is not present, that cell's activity becomes hampered or altered; if the deficiency continues, the cell suffers damage or disease—all the more reason to eat foods closer to nature.

Selective nutrition applies to the internal terrain as well. Blood and other bodily fluids nourish your cells, which make up your organs, which make up your systems, which are all connected. For instance, as you now know, your thyroid gland controls the metabolism of every cell in your body. Without enough iodine, thyroid activity slows down, affecting every cell and system—you get cold, tired, and constipated, your skin pales, and you may even develop large swellings called goiters. So can you imagine what happens when you're deficient in several minerals, vitamins, and phytochemicals?

Your terrain must have what it needs to influence your cells and glands in a healthy direction. You can't play cards with half a deck. Eating whole foods to obtain all their phytochemicals, known and unknown, is a necessity when you're balancing your terrain.

AMINO ACIDS

Amino acids are the building blocks of protein and are necessary for the growth and reproduction of all your cells. Any time your body is required to make something out of protein, the necessary amino acids are joined into chains called peptides, and the peptides are then combined to form protein molecules. Organs, blood vessels, muscle and other tissues, enzymes, and various hormones and neurotransmitters are made of specific combinations of amino acids; without them there would be no life.

Protein, when it's digested properly, breaks down into amino acids ready for absorption. Once absorbed, amino acids travel through specific pathways in the body to wherever they are needed. But we often don't eat the proper proteins, or we have poor digestion, or some proteins are destroyed by cooking, or we are enzyme-deficient—and any of these problems can lead to amino acid deficiencies. A single minor deficiency can easily affect certain metabolic pathways. A toxin can do the same thing, also resulting in amino acid deficiencies.

A metabolic pathway is like a road map; it is a course that a specific nutrient travels through the body. Along this pathway, it hooks up with other nutrients (vitamins, minerals, amino acids, and the like) to form a structure that is needed to repair or replace a tissue, hormone, antibody, or any number of things that may be required. This is a continuous process, so the necessary materials must always be present in the body.

The amino acid tryptophan, for example, must react with vitamin C and B$_6$ before it can be converted to serotonin, the neurotransmitter that relaxes you, guards against stress, and puts you to sleep at night. When these nutrients are destroyed by such things as overcooking or smoking foods or drinking alcohol excessively, the tryptophan-serotonin pathway is blocked, resulting in a deficiency in serotonin. Depression, insomnia, anxiety, and panic attacks are results of serotonin deficiency.

Amino Acid Therapy

If your digestive tract's pH is off-kilter and therefore you're not digesting protein properly, it doesn't matter how much protein you eat, because it won't be absorbed to be of any use. For that reason or any of the others noted above, your body may be lacking the amino acids that it needs. Free-form amino acid supplements, however, are mostly unaffected by the problems of food processing and inadequate digestion. Because they are predigested, they are quickly and easily absorbed. Taking singular or combined amino acids is called free-form amino acid therapy.

In any situation when you want to take amino acids, please have amino acid and mineral analyses done and get some professional advice. Reality Health Research offers a urine test that can determine what vitamins, minerals, and amino acids you may be deficient in. It is best to see your whole profile, because as you know, all nutrients work synergistically in the body. You or your doctor can consult with Reality Health Research (877-454-3313); they will suggest and even formulate supplements for your specific needs. If you prefer a blood test for an amino acid profile, have your licensed healthcare practitioner call Metametrix Clinical Laboratory for a test kit (770-446-5483).

Always use a combination of amino acids. Never take just one amino acid for a long period of time—more than two months—because that can cause a depletion of the others. For example, for phenylalanine to work, methionine must be present, and using only one of them will deplete the other, taking it away from its various functions in the body. This chapter discusses which ones to use together. If you want to use a particular amino acid for any length of time, I always suggest taking an amino acid supplement that contains all of the eight essential amino acids (described below), along with larger doses of the single amino acid of choice.

Amino acids come in three forms: D, DL, and L. The L forms are most easily absorbed and utilized, whereas the D forms must first be converted by the body. Usually B-vitamins and vitamin C are taken along with amino acids; vitamins can be combined with an amino acid product or taken separately. It's best to take amino acids in water or pineapple juice between meals on an empty stomach. Sometimes they cause constipation, so drink plenty of water and make sure you have adequate fiber daily to avoid any potential problem.

As you'll see, suggested doses of amino acids vary tremendously. In most situations, smaller doses are for longer periods of time and larger doses are for shorter periods (two weeks to two months). You can feel safe following the recommended dosage on the product's label, or you can consult your healthcare professional. Never take more than 1,000 milligrams of any amino acid in one day, unless you're working with an experienced practitioner who has given you the go-ahead.

Certain individuals must take special precautions in the use of amino acids. *Cautions:* Do not take phenylalanine if you are phenylketonuric. Phenylketonuria is an inherited condition in which people cannot metabolize phenylalanine properly; if people with phenylketonuria ingest phenylalanine, they get very sick. If you are taking monoamine oxidase inhibitors (MAOIs) or other antidepressants, avoid phenylalanine, tyrosine, and tryptophan, as these are precursors for the manufacture of stress hormones and serotonin, and an excessive surge of any of these could be problematic. If you can wean yourself off the antidepressants with your doctor's supervision, then it should be fine to take amino acids.

Meet Your Essential Amino Acids

Some books say there are twenty amino acids, and others say there are twenty-two. Experts agree, however, that there are eight essential amino acids and all others can be made from these eight. They're called essential because the body cannot manufacture them, so it's essential to take them in through food. The eight essential amino acids are phenylalanine, tryptophan, methionine, lysine, leucine, isoleucine, valine, and threonine.

Phenylalanine. After digestion, a certain amount of the phenylalanine you eat is used to make insulin. It also contributes to building the collagen structures in your skin and connective tissue. The body also converts some phenylalanine to the amino acid tyrosine (described below), and both are used to synthesize an important group of neurotransmitters and hormones called catecholamines. The catecholamines include L-dopa, dopamine, noradrenaline, and adrenaline. They prepare the body for fight-or-flight, increase alertness, and elevate mood. A deficiency in phenylalanine can cause anxiety, panic attacks, and depression.

Phenylalanine and tyrosine can be taken together for depression, stress, and low adrenal function. Phenylalanine is also helpful for weight control because it stimulates the intestines to secrete the hormone cholecystokinin, which signals the brain that you are full and satisfied. Additionally, phenylalanine helps relieve pain by inhibiting the breakdown of endorphins, which are naturally occurring short-chain amino acid molecules with potent analgesic activity, so the endorphins can continue circulating in the bloodstream.

Phenylalanine is found in foods such as meats, poultry, almonds, sesame seeds, and lentils. When supplementing, use the L or DL form for best results. The typical dose is 2–8 grams between meals. Larger doses are used for pain relief. *Note:* Do not take phenylalanine if you have high blood pressure or the condition called phenylketonuria.

Tyrosine. Although tyrosine is not technically an essential amino acid, I am including it here because of its partnership with phenylalanine (above). Tyrosine is a precursor to thyroid and adrenal hormones.

Tyrosine and iodine taken together have relieved symptoms of low thyroid and adrenal function, such as low body temperature and low blood pressure. Tyrosine has also been used to enhance the synthesis of dopamine, norepinephrine, and epinephrine; it is transported to catecholamine-secreting neurons in the adrenal glands where these neurotransmitters are manufactured.

Taking a drug doesn't replace the raw materials needed to produce neurotransmitters. Antidepressant drugs raise brain levels of serotonin and norepinephrine; using supplemental tyrosine, phenylalanine, and tryptophan is a safer and more natural way of doing this. Conversely, a deficiency in these three amino acids can cause depression, panic attacks, and anxiety. If you are experiencing any of these conditions, I recommend getting an amino acid profile done. You may be amazed how simply your problem can be solved. (I've never heard of a Prozac or Xanax deficiency.)

There are many food sources of tyrosine, including almonds, avocados, bananas, dairy products, lima beans, pumpkin seeds, and sesame seeds. When supplementing, suggested tyrosine dosages range from 500 milligrams to 2 grams daily.

Tryptophan. Tryptophan's primary role in the body is as a precursor to serotonin. (See the description of 5-HTP in the chapter on Choosing the Right Diet and Supplements.) Serotonin is a calming, relaxing neurotransmitter that relieves anxiety, panic, and depression. At night, the release of serotonin in the brain helps put you to sleep. Foods rich in tryptophan include oats and brown rice; red meat, eggs, fish, and poultry; bananas, mangoes, and dates; milk, yogurt, and cottage cheese; sunflower, sesame, and pumpkin seeds; and chickpeas, peanuts, spirulina, and chocolate.

B-vitamins, especially niacin, are needed for tryptophan to be metabolized properly. A dose of 2–8 grams of tryptophan along with B-vitamins and magnesium has produced positive effects for people who have anxiety, depression, or sleep disorders. A dose of 1,000 milligrams taken a half-hour before bedtime has done wonders for insomniacs. (*Sahley B, Birker KM. Heal with Amino Acids and Nutrients. Pain and Stress Publications, San Antonio, TX, 2001.*) Tryptophan can be taken in the daytime without producing sleepiness because the body uses it for other functions. *Caution:* People taking MAOIs should not use tryptophan.

Methionine. This sulfur-containing amino acid is called a methyl donor, as it is a source of the methyl molecules used in the synthesis of RNA and DNA. Methyl groups also bind with free radicals, making methionine an antioxidant.

Methionine is acted upon by enzymes to make the compound s-adenosyl methionine (SAMe); both have been used in the treatment of depression, suicidal tendencies, and intellectual sluggishness. SAMe increases the body's metabolism of L-dopa to the neurotransmitter dopamine and other catecholamines. (See the chapter on Choosing the Right Diet and Supplements.)

Methionine is also used in the body's production of cysteine; both of those compounds act as powerful detoxification agents capable of removing heavy metals from the body. In the conversion of methionine to cysteine, however, an intermediate compound called homocysteine is produced. If there is a deficiency of the B-vitamins folic acid, B_{12}, and B_6, the body's homocysteine level increases, increasing the risk of heart attack and stroke. Therefore, it's important to take these B-vitamins if your homocysteine level is higher than normal.

Methionine is found in foods such as beef, chicken, liver, sardines, pumpkin seeds, and lentils. Supplemental doses of methionine are 800–3,000 milligrams per day.

Lysine. Lysine is required in the formation of collagen, cartilage, and other connective tissues. It is also necessary for the body's synthesis of the vital compound carnitine. (Carnitine is detailed in the chapter on Choosing the Right Diet and Supplements.)

Recent research suggests that high doses of supplemental lysine and reduced dietary intake of arginine (described below) may be helpful in promoting the remission of recurring herpes outbreaks. (*Griffith RS. Success of L-lysine therapy in frequent recurrent herpes simplex infection. Determatologica 1987 175:183-190.*)

Food sources of this amino acid are red meat, pork, poultry, eggs, and certain fish (such as cod and sardines); nuts, soybeans and soy protein products, spirulina, and fenugreek seed; and cheese (particularly parmesan). The suggested supplement dosage for lysine is 300–1,200 milligrams.

Branched-chain amino acids (BCAAs). These three amino acids, leucine, isoleucine, and valine, work together in the body and are metabolized in the muscles instead of the liver. BCAAs comprise one-third of our muscle protein and are therefore of particular interest to athletes.

When taken before exercise, BCAAs affect the response of growth hormone, insulin, and testosterone, hormones that improve muscle mass, speed, strength, and agility. One study showed that taking BCAAs one to two hours before intense training decreased the breakdown of testosterone during the training period and increased testosterone levels afterward. (*Carli G, et al. Changes in the exercise-induced hormone response to branched chain amino acid administration. Eur J Appl Physiol 1992 64:272-277.*)

Muscles use BCAAs directly for energy, thereby sparing protein breakdown in the muscle tissue itself. This makes them an excellent energy source for distance runners, wrestlers, and anyone in endurance sports, as well as for body-builders. Leucine is used faster in the muscle than any other amino acid; even during moderate exercise, its oxidation rate increases by 240 percent.

BCAAs are found in all protein-rich foods, especially red meat, dairy products, eggs, whey protein, and legumes such as peanuts. The suggested supplement dosage for BCAAs is 1,000–3,000 milligrams daily.

Threonine. This essential amino acid serves as a carrier for phosphate in phosphoproteins. Threonine is also incorporated into other proteins and enzymes. People who are under stress need more threonine. Threonine can also be broken down into glucose for energy when needed.

Food sources of threonine include eggs, soy protein sources, seaweed, sesame seeds, cod, and certain cheeses. The suggested supplement dosage range for threonine is 1–5 grams daily.

Non-Essential Amino Acids

Although they are not termed "essential," the amino acids that can be synthesized by the body are nonetheless vital for optimal health. They can also be useful to athletes and exercisers as well as in certain disease states.

Histidine. Histidine is important to the immune system. In the body, histidine is converted into histamine and stored in the mast cells embedded within mucous membranes. When mast cells are attacked by viruses or bacteria, they burst and release histamine, which causes an inflammatory response with redness and swelling. Histidine is therefore a good amino acid to support immune functions and has been used therapeutically for allergic reactions. It is also a chelator of accumulated heavy metals, especially copper and iron.

As histidine tends to relax blood vessels, it has also been used to lower blood pressure and help with some cardiac conditions. However, in some patients, overloading with histidine may raise blood pressure, so low doses are advised. In their book *Life Extension,* Durk Pearson and Sandy

Shaw point out that the release of stored histamine is also a prerequisite for sexual arousal. For cases of low libido in both men and women, they suggest supplemental histidine along with niacin and vitamin B6, because those B-vitamins are necessary for histidine's utilization. *(Pearson D, Shaw S. Life Extension. Warner Books, New York, NY, 1982.)*

Histidine-rich foods are brewer's yeast, egg whites, fish, peanut flour, soybean meal, and wheat germ. The suggested supplement dosage range is 1,000–4,500 milligrams daily.

Gamma amino butyric acid (GABA). This amino acid functions as a neurotransmitter; it is found throughout the nervous system and is the most widely distributed neurotransmitter in the brain. GABA plays a major role in inhibiting anxiety and panic and is good for mood disorders. By filling brain receptor sites, GABA slows or blocks excitatory messages from other neurotransmitters and hormones. It inhibits rapid firing of nerve responses throughout the body and relaxes the muscles and mind.

As Candace Pert states, "GABA receptors are throughout the body and brain and play a major role in the stress-anxiety network." *(Pert CB. Molecules of Emotion. Simon and Schuster, New York, NY, 1997.)* Feelings of anxiety, fear, anger, grief, and depression are related to a brain structure called the amygdala, part of the limbic system connecting several other parts of the brain. Everything in the nervous system is connected, and when you become emotionally upset, it affects your body as well.

Just because you can't see an emotion doesn't mean it can't have a physical effect. We think and feel through our glands; we have receptor sites throughout our bodies, and whether the emotion is a calming one or an excitatory one, hormones are secreted accordingly and influence the whole body. As Pert says, "Emotions are the connection between the mind and body, and there is no separation between the two. Mind doesn't dominate the body, it becomes the body. Body and mind are one."

Dr. Michael Gerson describes it this way: "The body has two brains—one in the head and the other in the gut. Gastrointestinal disorders like colitis, irritable bowel syndrome, and diverticulitis originate from the gut's brain." Because your brain communicates with your digestive tract, any emotional upset can cause almost any digestive problem. When you experience fear, for example, it doesn't stay only in your brain—you feel tightness throughout your body. Whatever nutrients are involved during this hormonal blast (magnesium, calcium, and GABA, for instance) get used up, eventually creating deficiencies, so the bodily response becomes more dramatic over time. GABA is depleted by years of stress and poor eating habits. Effects of GABA deficiency are mental as well as physical: panic attacks, anxiety, fear, paranoia, and out-of-control emotions.

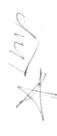

The brain can become deficient in needed substances just as any other part of the body can; prolonged anxiety alters brain chemistry. As athletes who over-train get worn out and deficient, they recover more slowly and become moody, depressed, and sluggish; when they rest and use good nutrition, they recover sooner. Why some professionals think the brain is any different is just old-fashioned training and refusal to change. They probably still wear bellbottoms and platform shoes, too.

Dr. Billie Sahley, a wonderful human being and founder of the Pain and Stress Clinic in San Antonio, Texas, states, "Twenty years of scientific evidence has shown that people with addictions have a deficiency of GABA, serotonin, glutamine, and other neurotransmitters. These deficiencies can be corrected by proper supplementation of needed neurotransmitters. No two people will have the same nutritional requirements." *(Sahley BJ. GABA: The Anxiety Amino Acid, 2nd ed. Pain and Stress Publications, San Antonio, TX, 2001.)*

Why then is the same drug prescribed for everyone for the same condition? Antidepressant drugs only help temporarily. Benzodiazepines such as Xanax, Lexotan, Valium, and Librium mimic GABA by attaching themselves to cell receptor sites in the brain. But as soon as you stop taking the drug, the symptoms return. If you are deficient in GABA or other amino acids, drug treatment does not address the cause. So people have to stay on these drugs, leading to more biochemical imbalance the longer the drugs are taken. Mood-altering drugs suppress our natural highs and lows, our true feelings. GABA and other amino acids, however, get to the root of the problem.

GABA is found in foods such as fish and wheat bran. The proper use of supplemental GABA is important. Usually a 500-milligram capsule dissolved in water three times a day is sufficient. A dose a half-hour before bedtime promotes relaxation and sleep. Nutrients that are used along with GABA are magnesium and the amino acids glutamine, taurine, and glycine (described below). Anyone who has panic attacks, anxiety, or related symptoms should investigate this group of nutrients and have an amino acid profile done to check for possible deficiencies. (In *The Great Anxiety Escape*, from Matulungin Publishing, Max Ricketts describes a nutritional program for anxiety, including GABA.)

Glutamine. Glutamine supports many functions in the human body and is an essential energy source for the intestines, immune system, and muscles. It was long considered a non-essential amino acid, but because of its importance, it is now considered a conditionally essential amino acid. Good food sources of glutamine include poultry, beef, fish, cabbage, beets, and dairy products.

During periods of stress and illness, muscle tissue is broken down to yield large quantities of glutamine, which are then carried to the kidneys, intestines, liver, and immune cells to aid in the repair process. One study showed that up to one-third of the amino acids released by the body's tissues at times of stress was glutamine, most of it from muscle breakdown. This is one of the reasons why the body degenerates during chronic illness, from what is called muscle wasting. Some healthcare professionals have recently begun giving glutamine to chronically ill patients.

The high concentration of glutamine in the blood is only one-thirtieth of the body's total. Its highest concentration is in muscle, which discharges glutamine into the bloodstream whenever it's needed. If a blood test reveals glutamine deficiency, it's likely that the muscle tissue is glutamine-deficient as well. However, a study measuring glutamine levels before and after surgery revealed that blood glutamine stayed constant, while muscle glutamine decreased 50 percent. *(Rennie MJ, et al. Skeletal muscle glutamine transport, intramuscular glutamine concentration. Metabolism 1989 38:47-51.)* This underscores the fact that blood tests don't give the entire picture. Tissues give up their nutrients to the blood for survival, so a deficiency at that point is difficult to detect. Tests have now been developed to determine the levels of nutrients within tissues, not simply what's present in the bloodstream.

Sickness and exercise are both stressors that can force the body into a catabolic state in which tissue breaks down and the internal terrain becomes acidic. Athletes and body-builders should be aware that exercise produces surplus acid; in response, the muscles send glutamine to the kidneys to help neutralize the acid. By monitoring your pH, you can tell if your terrain becomes too acidic, in which case it's a good idea to take extra glutamine while training to prevent muscle breakdown.

Intestinal cells use glutamine as their main source of energy as they rapidly grow and regenerate. During stress and illness, this activity increases dramatically, causing muscles to break down to release their glutamine for use in the intestinal cells' continual repair. In cases of leaky gut syndrome, taking extra glutamine along with probiotics promotes intestinal healing. Glutamine therapy has also been used for other gastrointestinal conditions including ulcers, diarrhea, inflammatory bowel disease, Crohn's disease, and colitis. Up to 40 grams of glutamine per day has been used in chronic conditions, but the usual dosage range is 5–15 grams per day. *(Shabert J, Ehrlich N. The Ultimate Nutrient: Glutamine. Avery Publishing Group, Garden City Park, NY, 1994.)*

Glutamine plays a role in your brain's well-being, as it is a precursor for the excitatory neurotransmitter glutamic acid and the inhibitory neurotransmitter GABA (described above). In one study, children's IQ test scores were found to increase when they were given glutamine. *(Rogers LL, Pelton RB. Effects of glutamine on IQ scores of mentally deficient children. Tex Rep Biol Med 1957 15:84-90.)* Another study giving 250–1,000 milligrams per day of glutamine to depressed individuals clearly demonstrated the amino acid's antidepressant properties. *(Cocchi R. Antidepressive properties of L-glutamine. Acta Psychiatr Belg 1976 76:658-666.)* In my practice, I have also seen clients recover from depression and anxiety by taking supplemental glutamine and GABA.

Caution: There are situations in which glutamine should only be used under a doctor's supervision, such as during liver or kidney disease or pregnancy. As I have mentioned, it's good to get an amino acid profile before any amino acid therapy is undertaken.

Taurine. This sulfur-containing amino acid is abundant in the heart, skeleton, muscles, and central nervous system. In the gall bladder, taurine combines with glycine and bile acids and has a protective effect against gall gladder disease. It is the second most important inhibitory neurotransmitter in the brain and functions in conjunction with glycine (described below) and GABA, which is why it has been used successfully for anxiety and as an anticonvulsant. Taurine has been shown to reduce potassium loss in heart muscle and is involved in regulating calcium transport in and out of cells. It is also used by the parathyroid gland to make a hormone called glutataurine.

Heart conditions, physical and emotional stress, and blood diseases cause large amounts of taurine to be lost in the urine. Low levels of this amino acid have been found in hypothyroidism, infertility, obesity, depression, and hypertension. Patients with these conditions may benefit from taking supplemental taurine. Clinicians at the Brain Bio Center in Rocky Hill, New Jersey report that taurine is also diminished in epileptic patients, and that supplemental taurine has been used successfully to treat many patients with seizure disorders. (*Murphy PA. Treating Epilepsy Naturally. McGraw-Hill, New York, NY, 2001.*)

Taurine is found in foods such as shellfish, fish, meat (especially organ meats), eggs, and milk. The range of effective supplementation dosage (relative to the particular condition) is 500–5,000 milligrams per day.

Glycine. Glycine is the third most important inhibitory neurotransmitter in the brain. In the spinal cord, it is involved in involuntary movements. It has been used—often along with B-vitamins—to help relieve spasms and contractions, relax the body during anxiety, and improve overall muscle tone. It does this by inhibiting abnormal responses from the spinal cord.

Glycine is involved in the body's production of DNA, phospholipids, and collagen. Glycine and arginine are highly concentrated in the skin and connective tissue and have been used in their healing. (*Minuskin ML. Nitrogen retention, muscle creatine and orotic acid excretion in traumatized rats fed arginine and glycine enriched diets. J Nutrition 1981 111:1265-1274.*)

It is of interest to both senior citizens and body-builders that doses of 4–8 grams of glycine have increased growth hormone levels. (*Kasai K, et al. Glycine stimulated growth hormone release in man. Acta Endocrinol 1980 93:283-286.*) Dr. Carl Pfeiffer and his colleagues report that two hours after 30 grams of glycine taken orally, growth hormone levels were ten times greater than baseline levels. They also describe finding low glycine levels in epileptic patients and depressed patients. (*Braverman E, et al. The Healing Nutrients Within, 2nd ed. Keats Publishing, New Canaan, CT, 1997.*)

In addition to stimulating the pituitary gland's release of growth hormone, glycine works with the hormone glucagon to raise blood sugar levels (see the Insulin chapter). This is important when you are working to stabilize your blood sugar, whether while training or experiencing sugar imbalances.

It's interesting to note that gelatin, a product used for many years to promote nail growth, is a good food source of this amino acid, as it is 33 percent glycine. The average adult dose is 3–5 grams per day.

Arginine. Although arginine is classified as a non-essential amino acid, it is absolutely essential when it comes to wound healing. Following any type of injury, arginine quickly goes to work in repairing the tissue.

There is a difference of opinion as to whether arginine stimulates the growth of the herpes virus. It is known, however, that the amino acid lysine (described above) suppresses the virus. Therefore, in cases of herpes, arginine should only be taken along with a larger amount of lysine, or ornithine (described below) should be substituted for arginine.

Arginine's breakdown in the body releases a simple gas called nitric oxide (NO), which plays a role in an array of body systems. Taking supplemental arginine increases levels of beneficial NO. A compound related to NO, the recently discovered arginine-derived nitric oxide (ADNO), is a multifaceted molecular marvel. ADNO scavenges free radicals, prevents cholesterol oxidation, regulates blood pressure by relaxing arteries, prevents platelets from clumping into dangerous clots, and helps promote erections in men who have erectile dysfunction.

In *Heal with Amino Acids and Nutrients*, Dr. Sahley describes the roles of arginine and NO in sexual function: "When sexual stimulation is present, the penile nerves transmit their signals, activating the enzyme that converts arginine into nitric oxide within the penis. The release of nitric oxide triggers the erection process. Arginine goes beyond Viagra's capability naturally." *(Sahley BJ. Heal with Amino Acids and Nutrients. Pain and Stress Publications, San Antonio, TX, 2001.)* Dr. Ronald Klatz reports giving fifteen patients—both men and women—2,800 milligrams of arginine for two weeks, with the result that all of the patients had renewed sexual performance. *(Klatz R. Grow Young with HGH. Harper Collins, New York, NY, 1997.)*

Many athletes are familiar with supplemental arginine, as it stimulates the pituitary gland to release growth hormone, improves performance and physique, burns fat, and tones muscle. *(Fried R, Merrell W. The Arginine Solution. Warner Books, New York, NY, 1999.)* The dosage for this purpose is usually 2 grams before exercise on an empty stomach and another 2 grams before bedtime. *Caution:* Arginine is not recommended for schizophrenics, because it has been known to aggravate symptoms.

Arginine-rich foods include carob, chocolate, coconut, dairy products, gelatin, meat, oats, wheat, and wheat germ, as well as peanuts, soybeans, walnuts, and their oils.

Ornithine. Ornithine is a precursor to the amino acids arginine, glutamine, and proline. It has similar effects to arginine when taken orally, so in many situations it is given in place of arginine. When two amino acids are known to have similar activity, it's a good idea to use both of them together or in a multi-amino acid combination. In *Life Extension*, Pearson and Shaw state that taking 1–2 grams of ornithine on an empty stomach at bedtime promotes the release of growth hormone. Food sources of ornithine include meat, fish, dairy products, and eggs.

Glutathione. Glutathione is actually a biological compound of three amino acids: cysteine, glutamic acid, and glycine. As an antioxidant, it acts outside of cells to neutralize the free radicals and lipid peroxidation that insult the body and accelerate aging (see the Free Radicals and Antioxidants chapter). As far back as 1964, glutathione was proven to be helpful in eliminating accumulated heavy metals from the body. It also aids the liver in detoxifying carcinogens and protects the liver from alcohol damage. Glutathione has been used in treating a wide variety of diseases.

Glutathione-rich foods include avocado, watermelon, asparagus, grapefruit, potato, acorn squash, strawberries, orange, tomato, cantaloupe, broccoli, okra, peach, zucchini, and spinach. When taken as a supplement, the suggested dosage is 500 milligrams daily. Glutathione should be taken in combination with other antioxidants.

Amino Acids, Hormones, and Hormone Replacement Therapy

You've read how being deficient in certain amino acids can alter your hormones and affect your immune system. As you get older, your hormone levels diminish and you age accordingly. You've learned, however, that you can use this book's self-monitoring system coupled with good nutrition to supply your body with the raw materials to manufacture the hormones and other substances that it needs to function at its best.

If you suspect endocrine problems, you can get a blood or urine test to check your hormone levels. Make sure to request the profile for these hormones: dehydroepiandrosterone (DHEA), progesterone, thyroid hormones, total and free estrogens, total and free testosterone, pregnenolone, insulin-like growth hormone (IGH-1), and melatonin. An amino acid profile is a good idea as well. You may also have adrenal and pituitary tests done. Quest Diagnostics in San Juan Capistrano offers these tests (949-728-4000), as do a number of other laboratories; your licensed healthcare practitioner can order them.

When hormone replacement therapy (HRT) is considered, Dr. David Brownstein recommends avoiding synthetic hormones and using natural hormones in combination. I suggest reading Dr. Brownstein's book, *The Miracle of Natural Hormones*, published by Medical Alternatives Press. He states, "Natural hormones when used appropriately will enhance one's health and will treat or even cure diseases, all without any appreciable side effects." *(Brownstein D. The Miracle of Natural Hormones, 3rd ed. Medical Alternatives Press, West Bloomfield, MI, 2003.)* Never take any hormone, however, until you've gotten your hormone levels tested first. You should have them repeatedly monitored while you're on HRT. And remember, this type of treatment is not meant to go on forever.

INSULIN'S CONNECTION TO DISEASE

Insulin is connected to many health problems including heart disease, high blood pressure, type I and II diabetes, obesity, elevated triglycerides, high cholesterol, and more recently recognized conditions such as Syndrome X, a collective term used to describe the new insulin-related symptoms that keep popping up nowadays. But the whole insulin issue really isn't that difficult to manage, especially if you use fewer carbohydrates in your diet, keep your terrain balanced, and reduce your toxic load. Toxins in the body increase or decrease certain hormonal outputs, eventually causing an organ's function or secretion to decline, and ultimately the affected organ will atrophy. This can happen, for example, to your adrenal glands, thyroid gland, and pancreas.

I want to tell you about insulin because the diseases it's related to are so common that you probably already know something about them. If you learn how to control your insulin secretions, you can experience immediate positive results. Plus, when you're working to reverse any disease process, controlling your blood sugar can result in a faster recovery.

Insulin is a hormone secreted by the pancreas and released into the bloodstream to prevent the blood sugar level from getting too high. On the outside of your body's cells, there is a protein that acts as a receptor for insulin. When your blood sugar rises after a meal, insulin tells your cells to absorb that excess sugar. Insulin does this by flowing over the receptors, thereby attaching to the outside of the cells, and then being taken into the cells.

If these receptors aren't working properly, however, the sugar (glucose) level in the bloodstream remains high, and the problems begin. Type II diabetes is a result of this scenario. This is why insulin injections are used to lower glucose levels. It's important to control glucose levels, not only because your muscles, brain, and retina use glucose as their main source of energy, but also because there is a danger of damage to your nerves, heart, and kidneys if these levels are too high or too low.

Carbohydrates including sugar, especially the sugars in cakes, honey, puddings, muffins, and the like, cause your blood glucose to rise after your food is digested. Carbohydrates such as the starch in potatoes have to be broken down into simpler sugars before they can pass through the digestive tract into the bloodstream and then into the cells. When the body does not have sufficient amylase for carbohydrate breakdown, carbohydrate metabolism can be affected. People with diabetes or other pancreatic problems often need enzyme supplements. If you use enzymes to aid digestion, be sure that your formula contains all four digestive enzyme families: lipase, protease, amylase, and cellulase must all be present to do the job. (See the Enzymes chapter.)

You now have an idea of what should happen after a carbohydrate meal or some type of sugar is consumed: amylase should ensure the breakdown of carbs into simple sugars, and insulin should direct the cells' uptake of these sugars from the bloodstream. But things can begin to go wrong after years of eating too many carbohydrates—pasta, other grain-based foods, and sweets—have required the pancreas to secrete insulin almost constantly.

Any organ or gland can get exhausted after prolonged overuse. Let's say that after years of burdening your pancreas with a high-carbohydrate diet, you eat and digest yet another high-carb meal, and the sugar passes into your bloodstream. Your pancreas secretes insulin, but the insulin receptors on your cells aren't functioning properly anymore, so the sugar stays in your blood. Your pancreas then secretes even more insulin in an attempt to jump-start the receptors, which finally, slowly, get the cells to absorb the sugar.

At this point, from that over-secretion, too much insulin remains in the blood, creating a condition called hyperinsulinism. The receptors now start to become insulin-resistant, which can begin to cause sub-clinical symptoms such as excessive thirst, fatigue, blurred vision, and dehydration. These symptoms may not yet be recognized by your doctor as a chronic condition, but you are experiencing a functional disorder, and this can be detected by a physician well-schooled in natural therapeutics.

The effects of a high-carb diet are becoming increasingly well known. Instead of saying that an insulin-resistance problem is genetic, we must consider the fact that we change our genes' expression by consuming too many carbohydrates. This is what is happening to our children today: When they are young, they have plenty of digestive enzymes and a strong pancreas that can handle excessive carbohydrates, plus they are more active. But when they get older and those factors change, you can see what the results will be. Years of heightened pancreatic secretions create a disease process and an exhausted pancreas.

It may surprise you to learn that coronary artery disease is not only related to diet but also to insulin specifically. Insulin does many things in the body, including stimulating the growth of smooth muscle cells in arterial walls. Too much insulin can cause a thickening of these walls that narrows the passageway. You may recall that fats called low-density lipoproteins (LDLs) in cell membranes are attacked and oxidized by free radicals. Insulin can also cause oxidation by coating the LDLs with sugar. This happens during an insulin-resistant state when excess sugar remains in the blood for a long time, and it results in oxidation damage to the cell membranes in arterial walls.

Patrolling cells called macrophages engulf the oxidized LDLs and the cholesterol attached to them, but then they start sticking to the walls, forming plaque deposits. Now the blood's cholesterol level is going up at the same time that the arteries are narrowing—and there are two more insulin-related processes to add to this scenario. Insulin happens to be the messenger that tells the kidneys to hold onto salt and water. As increasing amounts of fat, water, and salt are pushed through narrowing arteries, the blood pressure is going to rise. What's more, high levels of insulin drive magnesium out of the body—magnesium that normally relaxes the arterial walls and heart muscle and relieves hypertension, as well as soothing anxiety and helping with sleep.

Insulin, Fat, and Hormones

Guyton's *Textbook of Medical Physiology* explains that in the absence of insulin, not only is fat not stored in the fat cells of adipose tissue, but it is immediately released in the form of free fatty acids that can then be used for energy throughout the body by almost all of our cells. *(Guyton AC, et al. Textbook of Medical Physiology, 5th ed. W.B. Saunders, Philadelphia, PA, 1976.)* This scenario is what body-builders love to do: starve themselves of carbohydrates so the body burns fat for energy. The more muscle cells you have, the more fat you're going to burn, so weight lifting to increase muscle mass is always a good idea for people who are older and for people who want to get lean.

The flip side of this picture is excess insulin secretion. Under this influence, more glucose is stored in the liver as fat and in the muscles as glycogen. The fats in the liver are triglycerides, which are then transported through the bloodstream to be deposited in adipose tissues. The liver is a major storage place for fat, and if it becomes what is called a fatty liver, several of its vital functions are inhibited. If the body's cells become insulin-resistant and the pancreas secretes even more insulin to compensate, even more fat is stored. The result? The waist expands and the thighs get pudgy, and if this process keeps going, it leads to obesity.

The proper combination of amino acids and fats helps keeps your hormonal system in balance because they are the building blocks for hormone production. Cholesterol molecules are used to build sex hormones such as dehydroepiandrosterone (DHEA), estrogen, progesterone, testosterone, and aldosterone. Insulin causes the uptake of cholesterol and other fats as well as amino acids. So if the cells aren't taking up enough insulin, they aren't taking up enough of those hormonal building blocks either, potentially causing a hormonal imbalance. Men can become testosterone-deficient and women can become estrogen-deficient, for instance, which can even lead to developing characteristics of the opposite gender—and may be dangerous if it continues for too long.

The Solution to Insulin Problems

You've now learned that if you are insulin-deficient or insulin-resistant, or have hyperinsulinism, all kinds of symptoms can arise. You've learned (again) that a group of seemingly unrelated symptoms may be caused by one thing: in this case, too many carbohydrates. Although the symptoms can be confusing, once they're understood, the solution can be simple. The development of these insulin-related problems is a good example of a normal bodily process disrupted. And you know by now that if you change an unhealthy process, you'll change the symptoms.

The key here is to lower your carbohydrate intake, which will reduce your insulin secretion. Over a period of time, your cells' receptors will become insulin-sensitive again, and everything can get back to normal. Reducing insulin secretion also lowers your cholesterol and triglyceride levels, and at the same time, your body begins to burn more fats for energy, which is a major key to weight loss. Decreasing insulin production also slows the aging process.

Grains and grain products, other starches, and sugars have a few things in common. They are all converted by digestion into glucose, triggering the insulin secretion that can result in weight gain and other significant health problems. Remember, these types of simple carbohydrates, if not utilized quickly by the body, are stored as fat. The complex carbohydrates in vegetables and fruits, however, produce a very different effect. Complex carbohydrates cause a slower release of glucose from the digestive tract into the bloodstream, largely because of the fiber content in these foods. Also, the vitamins and minerals they contain assist with the body's absorption and utilization of glucose and other nutrients.

With this smaller and more gradual increase in your blood sugar level after eating, your insulin secretions are released in smaller amounts over a longer period of time—so they don't produce the physical and emotional highs and lows caused by eating more concentrated carbohydrates and sugars. Therefore, the complex carbohydrates found in non-starchy vegetables, greens, and fruits can be the core of your diet. Eliminate simple carbohydrates, which are found in grains and grain products, potatoes, corn, soda, pasta, sugar, and all other sweeteners.

This book is not about the treatment of specific diseases, so my dietary suggestions for insulin-related conditions are not complete. But by now you're adding things up: you're increasing your antioxidant intake, checking for heavy metals, changing your diet, and working on balancing your terrain. You have a real handle on some of the causes of disease and you believe that you can do something about your health problems. Congratulations on your new understanding and progress! Even if you're not ill in any way, you can always be healthier and more helpful to others.

The Other Side of the Coin: Glucagon

The islets of Langerhans in the pancreas produce another hormone, glucagon, which is rarely talked about. Glucagon counterbalances the effect of insulin on blood sugar by causing glycogen in the liver to be broken down into glucose. That glucose is then dumped from the liver into the bloodstream, so the blood glucose level rises again just a few minutes after the secretion of glucagon.

Whenever the blood glucose level falls, the pancreas pours glucagon into the blood to rapidly bring blood glucose back up to normal. Thus, glucagon acts as a limiting system to prevent hypoglycemia, which is a blood glucose level that's too low. For example, when you eat large amounts of sugar, your pancreas secretes insulin, which activates the cells to absorb glucose from the blood. Most of the time, glucose is taken up so fast that a low blood sugar level results, so the pancreas then secretes glucagon to counterbalance. But that pancreatic balancing mechanism can get stressed, and even burned out, because of an endocrine response that connects a high-carb/high-sugar diet, the adrenal glands, and the pancreas, as described in the next section.

Diet, Stress, and the Endocrine System

Exercise is good—but serious exercise can exhaust your endocrine glands if you don't support them with good nutrition. I work with college athletes who are in excellent condition, but their urine and saliva are always acidic. This acidic state diminishes minerals, and sooner or later a big crash will come. If you're always acidic and low in minerals, what do you think the future will bring? Pain. Fortunately, the monitoring system can help you prevent this by telling you what your body needs to keep up the pace of your lifestyle.

Who would have thought that exercise and physical or psychological stress has a similar effect on the body as a high-carb, high-sugar, junk-food diet? As it turns out, a high-carb or sugary meal and strenuous exercise produce similarly acidic pH readings—and it doesn't stop there.

Here's what happens: you eat a high-sugar or grain-based meal, and the carbs and sugar are converted to a load of glucose that is rapidly absorbed into the bloodstream, creating a high blood glucose level. The pancreas immediately secretes insulin to signal the cells to absorb all this glucose, and then it secretes glucagon to counterbalance the insulin and restore blood sugar to normal. The problem is that when the blood and cells get blasted with this over-abundance of glucose, the pancreas overdoes its secretions. The result is a temporary "sugar high," and then you crash and feel dull and lethargic. Welcome to hypoglycemia.

Next, other glands and organs get involved. Because your heart, brain, and lungs require glucose for energy, your hypothalamus responds to your low blood sugar level by quickly signaling your pituitary gland to secrete adrenocorticotropic hormone (ACTH). ACTH travels via the bloodstream to your adrenal glands, stimulating them to secrete cortisol and adrenaline. Your liver responds to these hormones by converting amino acids into glucose and dumping it into the blood; similarly, your muscles give up their stored glucose to the blood.

Thanks to all of that compensation for your low blood sugar level, you start to feel better. But that glucose in your muscles was needed for muscle activity, and those amino acids were needed for ongoing tissue building and repair—so your body is "stealing from Peter to pay Paul." And now there is excess glucose in the bloodstream once again (unless it's promptly absorbed by the cells and burned for energy).

If this pattern continues, the pancreas weakens, the adrenals become overactive and secrete too much cortisol, and too much cortisol in the blood causes anxiety and insomnia. During excessive adrenal activity, blood pressure can rise; this is the high before the low, because when the adrenals are exhausted, low blood pressure results. (You'll be able to observe all of this with the monitoring system.) Meanwhile, the overactive adrenals are also secreting the hormone aldosterone, which signals your kidneys to reabsorb sodium, increasing blood volume and pressure. And any time the kidneys retain more sodium, the buffering minerals potassium and magnesium are lost in the urine.

When the body is undergoing emotional stress or a physical stress such as exercise, it holds onto more sodium to keep up the blood volume and pressure. This is a part of the "fight-or-flight" response, which is the body's built-in mechanism for self-preservation by kicking into high gear when confronted by, for example, a wild animal—or nowadays, an emergency at work, or a strenuous work-out. This response was described by Dr. Hans Selye in *The Stress of Life,* and it is essentially the same sequence of endocrine responses described above for the high-carb meal, starting with the hypothalamus and leading to the adrenals. *(Selye H. The Stress of Life. New York, NY, McGraw-Hill, 1978.)*

With all of those glands overworking in reaction to a perceived stressor, sodium is reabsorbed to retain water and constrict the blood vessels, because that will ensure a sufficient blood volume and pressure for the lungs, heart, brain, and muscles to perform during this excited state. No wonder people have heart attacks during stressful periods or events. Potassium and magnesium are lost in the urine as part of this same reaction, because they are vasodilators that would relax the blood vessels. When the body is assuming a defensive position, it does not want to relax. It does not distinguish between a highly emotional state, exercise, and a high-carbohydrate diet—it simply goes straight into fight-or-flight mode.

So whether you're angry, eating a high-carb meal, or lifting weights, the physiological end-point is the same: burnout and rapid aging. The difference between the stress reaction, the exercise reaction, and the high-carb reaction is that for exercise or stress, cortisol is secreted before insulin, whereas after a high-carb meal, insulin is secreted before cortisol as a direct response to the glucose in the blood, not as the result of a hormone's activity. But the results of all three reactions are the same, as illustrated below (a picture really can be worth a thousand words):

The Similar Effects of a High-Carb Diet and Stress

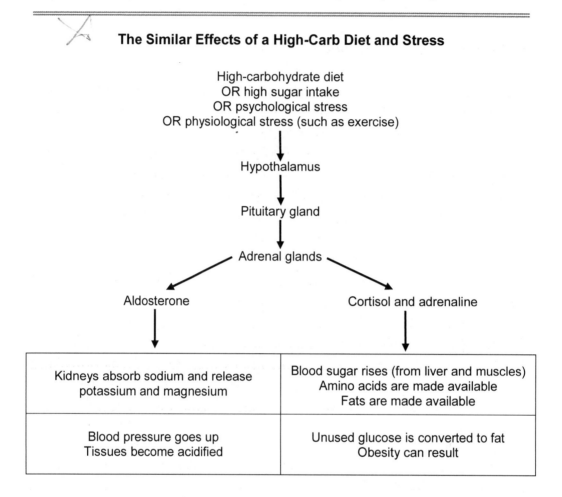

High-carbohydrate diet
OR high sugar intake
OR psychological stress
OR physiological stress (such as exercise)

↓

Hypothalamus

↓

Pituitary gland

↓

Adrenal glands

Aldosterone   Cortisol and adrenaline

Kidneys absorb sodium and release potassium and magnesium	Blood sugar rises (from liver and muscles) Amino acids are made available Fats are made available
Blood pressure goes up Tissues become acidified	Unused glucose is converted to fat Obesity can result

You usually have some extra glucose in your blood because your organs and cells seldom need all of it at any given moment. That's not a problem if excess sugar is released slowly from the digestive tract or from elsewhere in the body into the bloodstream, but that's not what's happening in the situations described above. And ultimately, that excess sugar gets turned into fat and stored in fat cells, leading to a syndrome of weight gain and eventual obesity.

Balancing Your Blood Sugar and Your Terrain

A little stress is actually a good thing for the body—exercise, after all, is a stress that benefits the muscles, nervous system, circulation, and more. But too much stress from any source, whether it's your diet or other aspects of your life, speeds aging and disease processes. Fortunately, using the monitoring system helps you determine when your body needs your attention to bring it back into balance and keep it there.

If you get a high blood pressure reading (increased adrenal activity), or urinary and salivary pH readings that are always in the acidic range, this indicates that your body is coping with some kind of stress. Low temperature (reduced thyroid activity) with low blood pressure (reduced adrenal activity) indicates low energy in your system. If you have low blood pressure, low temperature, and acidic pH readings, get to work on balancing your terrain, because this is the picture of total exhaustion.

The Glycemic Index (GI) rates how fast carbohydrates break down and increase blood sugar. It's best to choose foods that will raise your blood sugar less rapidly, thereby preventing an extreme insulin response (see graph below).

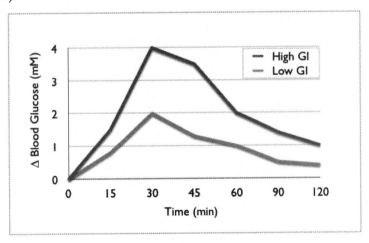

It's best to select foods in the low-to-medium GI range most of the time. After exercise, though, it's usually okay to eat foods that are higher on the chart. (For more information on the GI, see www.glycemicindex.com.)

Glycemic Ratings: L = Low, M = Medium, H = High, VH = Very High

Fruits and Vegetables

Food	GI	Serving	Carbs
Apple	L	1 each	25g
Asparagus	L	1 cup	8g
Banana	H	1 each	27g
Broccoli	L	1 cup	5g
Brussels sprouts	L	1 cup	8g
Cantaloupe	M	½ (5" diam.)	21g
Celery	L	1 stick	1g
Cherries	L	10	11g
Cucumber	L	6 slices	1g
Grapefruit	L	½ medium	9g
Grapes	M	20 medium	8g
Green beans, ckd.	L	1 cup	9g
Green pepper	L	1 each	5g
Lettuce	L	1 cup shred.	2g
Mushrooms	L	½ cup sliced	2g
Onion	L	1 cup sliced	10g
Orange	M	1 each	15g
Orange juice	M	6 ounces	20g
Peach	M	1 each	10g
Pear	M	1 each	25g
Pineapple, fresh	M	1 cup	19g
Plum	L	1 each	9g
Raisins	H	½ cup	66g
Spinach, cooked	L	1 cup	7g
Spinach, raw	L	1 cup	2g
Strawberries	L	1 cup	10g
Tomato	L	1 each	6g
Watermelon	M	1 cup	12g
Zucchini	L	1 cup	4g

Starches

Food	GI	Serving	Carbs
Applesauce	M	½ cup	14g
Bagel	H	1 whole	30g
Bread	H	1 slice	11g
Bread, wholegrain	H	1 slice	14g
Bread, reduced cal.	H	1 slice	6g
Carrots, cooked	H	½ cup	8g
Cereal, corn flakes	VH	1 ¼ cups	24g
Cereal, raisin bran	VH	1 ¼ cups	52g
Corn, on cob	H	1 ear	19g
Corn, cooked	H	1 cup	41g
English muffin	H	1 each	30g
Granola	H	1 cup	67g
Hamburger bun	H	1 each	26g
Kidney beans	H	1 cup	40g
Muffin, bran	H	1 each	30g
Oatmeal, cooked	M	1 cup	25g
Pasta, cooked	M	1 cup	40g
Peas	M	1 cup	25g
Pita bread	M	1 each	23g
Pinto beans	M	½ cup	22g
Popcorn, popped	VH	1 cup	6g
Potato	H	1 baked	51g
Pretzels	H	10 sticks	4g
Refried beans	M	½ cup	24g
Rice	H	1 cup	40g
Rice cakes	VH	1 each	8g
Roll, dinner	H	1 each	20g
Rye bread	M	1 slice	12g
Rye crackers	M	2	8g
Sweet potato/yam	M	1 med.	32g
Tortilla, corn	H	1 (6" diam.)	13g

In conjunction with these choices, monitor your salivary and urinary pH to see the effect that the foods have on your terrain. Some may make you acidic, others may alkalize you, and you can also try mixing foods to balance their effects. To evaluate the effect of a particular food or meal, take your pH readings before eating, wait two hours after eating, and take them again. If you spend some time with the monitoring system, you can design a healthy diet that puts less stress on your endocrine system.

A product from Moss Nutrition, Bio Adaptogen, helps normalize high or low cortisol levels; another product, Glucostate, is used for blood sugar control (have your licensed healthcare practitioner call 800-851-5444). But first, try using the monitoring system and making dietary adjustments to balance your terrain. Then, if necessary, add one supplement at a time. Wait a week, and then, if necessary, add another one.

The amino acids that your body uses for energy are glutamine, leucine, isoleucine, and valine. If your system is showing any indication of exhaustion, it's good to add these to your nutrition program. Take them on an empty stomach (between meals) with water or pineapple juice. Any time you use free-form amino acids, it helps to take them along with B-vitamins and vitamin C (Juice Plus+® is an excellent source) to aid their absorption and proper metabolism. If you're undecided about which amino acids to take, use a multiple amino acid complex, particularly if you aren't digesting protein properly. I recommend Aminoplex from Mountain States Health Products (800-MHP-0074).

Earlier in this book, you learned about the minerals that act as the buffering system to neutralize acids in the bloodstream. Now you know how those minerals are affected by a high-carb diet or by stress. As you become more acidic over a period of time, you become mineral-deficient, influencing the function and health of all your glands, organs, and tissues. Becoming acidic through exposure to environmental chemicals and heavy metals, in addition to eating a diet full of carbohydrates, acid-producing foods, and the wrong fats, leads you into chronic disease.

Chromium is particularly helpful in the control of insulin and blood sugar levels. Chromium increases the attachment of insulin to cell walls, facilitating the passage of blood sugar into the cells. In the brain, this process also helps turn off hunger when sugar gets into the brain cells that control appetite. When you are chromium-deficient, however, insulin is less efficient, so wide swings in blood sugar can result, and the sugar not utilized as fuel is converted to fat and stored—plus, the appetite-control center isn't turned off properly, so hunger persists and you get unnatural food cravings. Chromium is usually taken in the form of chromium picolinate.

FATS AND YOUR TERRAIN

Using the proper fats is very important when you are balancing your terrain. In this chapter, you will learn which fats are good for you and which ones can negatively affect your body. Specific fats, for instance, have antifungal, antibacterial, antiviral, antioxidant, and anti-inflammatory qualities. Certain oils and fatty acids are excellent for your cardiovascular system. On the other hand, it's very difficult to balance your terrain or recover from a chronic condition while using rancid and toxic oils. Beware of frying foods with vegetable oil, which creates free radicals. As you read earlier, free radicals cause lipid peroxidation, which can initiate plaque buildup in your blood vessels.

Polyunsaturated oils are very vulnerable to attack by free radicals, causing tissue damage and excess lipid peroxidation, which increases acidification in your tissues. Hydrogenated oils inhibit cells' oxygen uptake, diminish the normal flow of electrolytes in and out of cells, damage cell membranes, and cause cell leakage. Once its membrane is damaged, the cell's immunity is impaired, as is its protection against bacteria and fungus. As you know, fungus (including yeast) secretes mycotoxins, which are deadly to cellular structures and create an acid residue. Using certain fatty acids, however, can prevent this.

Accumulated heavy metals can upset your internal terrain by destroying enzymes and fatty acids as well as by damaging cell membranes. Fatty acid deficiencies can have negative health consequences. Your cells must have the right fatty acids present for repair. If you have been exposed to heavy metals or have silver fillings (which are 45–50 percent mercury), it's a good idea to get checked for metal toxicity. A test kit to evaluate your fatty acid levels is available from Metametrix (your licensed healthcare practitioner can order this at 800-221-4640).

Essential Fatty Acids

Fatty acids are the primary components or building blocks of fats. Several of these are classified as essential fatty acids (EFAs) because our body cannot manufacture them, so it is essential that we get them through our foods. Two of the most important EFAs are alpha-linolenic acid (LNA) and linoleic acid (LA).

A deficiency in LA can produce symptoms such as hair loss, liver and kidney degeneration, mental disturbances, hormonal deficiency, eczema, slow wound healing, sterility, miscarriages, sore joints, and heart and circulatory problems. Symptoms of LNA deficiency include general weakness, poor vision, learning disabilities, lack of motor coordination, behavioral changes, high blood pressure, edema (swelling), tissue inflammation, and low metabolic rate.

EFAs do not aggregate (clump together) in the blood unless they have been structurally altered or if your terrain has become toxic. They carry cellular wastes and other toxins through the bloodstream to the kidneys, intestinal tract, and lungs for elimination. They also give us mental vitality. They carry oxygen to all the cells in the body, including brain cells, so food can be burned for energy production.

LA is involved in hemoglobin production. It also helps hold protein in place in cell membranes, and thus helps control the passing of nutrients and fluid in and out of the cells through these protein "doors."

EFAs are also used by the body as precursors for building a family of hormone-like structures called prostaglandins. Prostaglandins control certain cellular functions, lower blood pressure, and inhibit other fats from sticking together in the blood. The brain, retina, inner ear, adrenal glands, and testicles all need prostaglandins that are produced from LNA and LA. At levels of 12–15 percent of our total caloric intake, EFAs increase the metabolic rate and thus increase the burning of calories that is so necessary for weight loss. The diet should contain approximately 3–6 grams of EFAs daily to avoid deficiencies; this amount can be increased for people who are healing from an injury or recovering from an illness, fatigue, or excessive stress.

EFAs are also part of the membranes of the tiny organelles inside cells, such as the endoplasmic reticulum where protein synthesis takes place and the mitochondria where fuel is burned (oxidized). EFAs are also found in the nucleus of the cell, where cellular functions including growth and repair are controlled. In children, LNA is required for brain development. Think how an LNA deficiency can affect mental acuity, growth of the brain, and also depression and anxiety in adults...

Most of us have never considered EFAs and the role they play in recovery from intense exercise or in various conditions such as chronic fatigue syndrome. They actually shorten the post-exercise recovery period and facilitate the conversion of lactic acid to water and carbon dioxide. LNA in particular speeds healing and increases stamina and vitality, which are important for recovery from any type of fatigue.

As hormone replacement therapy (HRT) is becoming a popular fix-it program, it's important to note that EFAs are the building blocks of sexual hormones. If you consume sufficient amounts of EFAs, you may not become hormone-deficient. Give your body the raw materials that it needs. When you take a particular hormone, the gland that naturally secretes that hormone may stop producing it.

If your doctor feels that HRT is necessary, combine it with EFAs and other nutrients, and you may then be able to ease off of HRT. Interesting research published recently in a French medical journal has shown that taking estrogen can increase women's risk of contracting cancer, and also that it doesn't protect against heart disease. *(Boissel JP, Cornu C. Pharmacology of estrogens and progestogens and cardiovascular risk. Therapie 1999 54:387-392.)* We'd better catch up with what the rest of the world is learning about the prevention of chronic diseases—more people die because of lack of knowledge than from anything else.

The Forms of Fats

All fats are made up of carbon, hydrogen, and oxygen. These are the same elements that compose carbohydrates, but the relative hydrogen content of fats is much higher. There are many types of fat, categorized by their various amounts of these elements and the different structures of their molecules.

We will consider two major groups of fats: saturated and unsaturated. The fundamental difference between saturated and unsaturated fats is the ratio of hydrogen to carbon. The unsaturated group is subdivided into polyunsaturated and monounsaturated fats.

Saturated fats. Saturated fats are the simplest. They are made up of carbon atoms hooked together in a chain, with each carbon atom attached to a hydrogen atom. Because each carbon has a hydrogen partner clinging to it, none of the carbons can take on another partner, so the fat is said to be saturated. These are usually found in animal foods such as beef, pork, and dairy products. Saturated fats are solid at room temperature, with melting points at higher temperatures than other fats.

Unsaturated fats. These fats have one or more carbon atoms in the chain that are not attached to hydrogen atoms. Because those carbons do not have hydrogen partners, these fats are called unsaturated (they are not "saturated" with hydrogen atoms). Unsaturated fats have one or more double bonds between those un-partnered carbons and a kink at the double-bond position. They are all negatively charged, which means that they repel each other and therefore do not stick together.

Unsaturated fats are usually of a more liquid consistency and can go rancid much faster than saturated fats. They have lower melting points, break up and disperse much more readily, and do not aggregate in the bloodstream. Unsaturated fats can also move easily within the cell membrane, and this fluidity makes it easier for them to transport nutrients and oxygen into the cell.

Polyunsaturated fats. Polyunsaturated fats have more than one double bond in their carbon chains. There are many different kinds; some are healthful and others are harmful. The polyunsaturated fats in refined and hydrogenated oils, for instance, are some of the worst! The heating and refining process actually alters them in such a way that they become destructive to human tissues. The healthful ones are also called natural polyunsaturated fats. (Technically, natural polyunsaturated fatty acids are called cis fatty acids, because their molecules are in what's called a cis configuration, in which both of the hydrogen atoms next to the carbon-carbon double bond are on the same side of the molecule. This cis configuration is the molecule's normal structure, in contrast to the unnatural trans configuration, discussed later in this chapter.)

Monounsaturated fats. These fats have only one double bond; that is, two of the carbons in the chain are double-bonded to each other and therefore lack two hydrogen partners. Because of the structural kink at the site of the double bond, monounsaturated fats don't stick together as easily as saturated fats, and therefore stay liquid at room temperature. But because they have only one double bond, they don't go rancid easily.

Polyunsaturated versus Saturated Fats in Diet and Disease

Most polyunsaturated fats are found in vegetable oils. The more carbon-carbon double bonds an unsaturated fat has, the more kinks there are in its molecular structure, and therefore the more liquid it is, because the kinks mean the molecules don't clump together much. Because there are reactive unpaired electrons at the double bond sites, polyunsaturated fats go rancid easily, and are damaged by sunlight and cooking. Spoiling and damage make unsaturated oils unsuitable to consume.

As Udo Erasmus describes in *Fats that Heal, Fats that Kill:* "Light, the greatest enemy of EFAs, produces free radicals in oils and speeds up the reaction of oils with oxygen from the air by 1,000 times, resulting in toxic, rancid fatty acids. Light destroys the healthy properties of EFAs and breaks them down into aldehydes and ketones." *(Erasmus U. Fats that Heal, Fats that Kill. Alive Books, Burnaby, BC, Canada, 1993.)* Aldehydes (you've heard of formaldehyde) and ketones are harmful chemicals.

The information we have been given about saturated fats being bad for us and polyunsaturated fats being good for us is wrong. We have only been given half-truths. It's not the saturated fats we should be avoiding— it's the rancid and overcooked polyunsaturated fats and oils that are creating free radical damage.

Polyunsaturated fats are loaded with free radicals after they are cooked or go rancid, and therefore can cause damage at the cellular level anywhere in the body—they attack red blood cells and damage DNA and RNA, blood vessels, and skin. And as you've learned, free radical damage initiates the buildup of plaque in your arteries. As it turns out, excess consumption of polyunsaturated fats has been linked to cancer, heart disease, digestive diseases, and problems in reproductive organs.

Meanwhile, saturated fats constitute 50 percent of the cell membrane, protect the liver from alcohol and other toxins, enhance immune system function, and must be present for the body's proper utilization of EFAs. Long-chain saturated fatty acids surround the heart to provide insulation and protect it from free radical damage. Some short-chain saturated fatty acids have helpful antimicrobial and antifungal properties. But don't be mistaken: if any fat, saturated or unsaturated, is overly cooked or processed to the point that its molecular structure is altered and damaged, it can wreak havoc in the body.

Is an extremely low-fat diet the answer? You've probably heard of Nathan Pritikin's low-fat diet. When people on his diet lost weight and lowered their cholesterol levels, these benefits were believed to be due to the reduction of dietary fat, even though Pritikin made several other significant recommendations: to consume more fresh fruits and vegetables, and to eliminate sugar, processed foods, white flour, alcohol, coffee, tobacco, and salt.

Pritikin's diet was 5–10 percent fat, 10–15 percent protein, and 80 percent complex carbohydrates. It soon became apparent that those people who could manage to stay on it experienced a variety of health problems such as poor concentration, depression, vitamin and mineral deficiencies, and premenstrual syndrome (PMS). Researchers have since shown that such an extremely high-carb diet can also lead to other problems if maintained over a long period of time. (Read Ann Louise Gittleman's book *Beyond Pritikin,* from Bantam Books, in which she explains the pitfalls of a low-fat, high-carb diet—she worked at the Pritikin Longevity Center.)

Consider by contrast the Eskimos of Greenland, who eat a diet that is 70 percent fat and yet have an extremely low incidence of heart disease and cancer. The key is the source and types of this fat. The Eskimos eat seals, whales, walrus, and fatty coldwater fish such as herring, mackerel, and salmon. These marine foods contain oils high in two omega-3 fatty acids: eicosapentaenoic acid (EPA) and docosahexaenoic acid (DHA), both of which protect the cardiovascular system.

We have been told that we should decrease our intake of fats, particularly saturated fats from animal products, and that their cholesterol causes heart disease. Those recommendations are now being questioned; you'd be surprised to learn that there is very little evidence to support them. But there is plenty of evidence demonstrating that the real demons are vegetable oils, processed oils and fats, hydrogenated oils, and the free radical damage done by these fats inside the body and even outside on the surface of the skin. As you recall, the peroxidation of LDL is a significant factor in circulatory and heart disease.

Before 1920, heart disease was rare, but the incidence of coronary heart disease rose dramatically in the ensuing forty years. Today heart disease is responsible for 40 percent of all deaths in the United States. At the same time, consumption of sugar and processed foods increased by 60 percent, and consumption of vegetable oils and refined oils rose a tremendous 400 percent. (Research like this can be found in books such as Mary Enig's *Know Your Fats*, from Bethesda Press, and *Trans Fatty Acids in the Food Supply*, from Enig Associates.)

Numerous studies have shown that eating cholesterol and a high-fat diet is not, in fact, related to heart disease. One study found that Jews in Yemen, whose dietary fats were solely of animal origin, had a lower incidence of heart disease than Yemenite Jews living in Israel, whose diet contained vegetable oils and margarine. A similar study found that the people of Northern India ate seventeen times more animal fat than the people of Southern India but had seven times less coronary artery disease. (*Malhotra S. Indian J Industrial Med 1968 14:219.*) Another study, published as *The Long-Living of Soviet Georgia*, revealed that the people in that part of the former Soviet Union who ate the most meat lived the longest. (*Pitskhelauri GZ. The Long-Living of Soviet Georgia. Human Sciences Press, New York, NY, 1982.*) And since World War II, the Japanese have increased their consumption of animal fat and their life span has increased as well.

When I visited France, I found the French diet to be loaded with cream, cheese, and other saturated fats—yet France has less heart disease than the United States. That has been attributed to the French drinking red wine, but no amount of red wine would offset the amount of saturated fat they consume, so saturated fat can't be the real culprit in heart disease. You'd think we would have come to this conclusion once we discovered that mother's milk is 50 percent fat, most of it saturated. (Commercial baby formulas, however, are low in fat and cholesterol, which are both needed for proper hormone production and brain development.)

Cholesterol Myths by Uffe Ravnskov is very enlightening on this subject. In a nutshell, we have been told that the amount of fat and cholesterol we eat makes our blood cholesterol level go up and causes heart disease. Unfortunately, conclusions are often drawn from insignificant studies or results slanted toward profit-oriented special interest groups. Research studies do not consistently demonstrate a significant correlation between saturated fat consumption and heart disease.

In England, for example, the incidence of heart attacks increased tenfold from 1930 to 1970, but saturated fat consumption in England did not increase during that 40-year period. *(Yudkin J. Diet and coronary thrombosis: hypothesis and fact. Lancet 1957 2:155-162.)* Famed heart surgeon Michael DeBakey surveyed 1,700 patients who had atherosclerosis, or hardening of the arteries, and found no relationship between blood levels of cholesterol and the incidence of atherosclerosis. *(Garrett HE, et al. Serum cholesterol values. in patients treated surgically for atherosclerosis. JAMA 1964 189:655-659.)*

One of the largest and most frequently cited studies on risk factors for heart disease is the Framingham Heart Study involving over 6,000 people (www.framinghamheartstudy.org). It is quoted by the authors of all the magazines and books that still claim that animal fats are the problem. However, the director of that very study states that the more saturated fat, cholesterol, and calories the participants ate, the lower their serum cholesterol was. It was also found that the more of these fat-containing foods they ate, the more active they were and the less they weighed.

If animal fat and high blood cholesterol are the villains, then eating less of these should logically cause a significant decrease in cholesterol levels and heart disease, right? Well, I haven't seen studies that consistently demonstrate this result. In fact, some studies, including the Framingham study, have shown that above the age of forty-seven, cholesterol levels make no difference at all in the likelihood of having heart disease.

Nowadays, we do know that smoking, high insulin levels, high carbohydrate and sugar consumption, stress, free radical damage, chlorinated water, hydrogenated oils, and the like increase cholesterol and increase risk of heart disease. Yet when you read most studies of dietary risk factors and heart disease, most of those factors are not even considered. I encourage you to do your own research in this area. (A good source on the subject is www.thincs.org.)

The "Mediterranean diet" is alleged to be a low-fat, mainly vegetarian diet resulting in less heart disease. You've got to be kidding me—in which Mediterranean country do people live on a vegetarian diet? I'm Italian. Italians eat cheese, eggs, fish, meatballs... Don't even think about giving me a tofu meatball. And it's the same with the Greeks. The saturated fat content in the Mediterranean diet is surprisingly higher than most people realize. But once you replace natural foods with processed foods, a high-carb/high-sugar diet, and bad oils—now you've got heart disease.

Forms of Fatty Acids

All saturated, polyunsaturated, and monounsaturated fats and oils are combinations of fatty acids. The number of carbons hooked together determines whether they are short-chain, medium-chain, or long-chain fatty acids. These three groups of fatty have different characteristics, sources, and uses.

Short-chain fatty acids. These are usually saturated because they contain only three to twelve carbon atoms and fewer carbon-carbon double bonds than are found in longer chains. Butterfat from cow's milk and goat's milk are examples. Short-chain fatty acids contribute to your health by being antimicrobial and supporting your immune system. They are found in coconut oil, butter, and palm kernel oil and have a much higher melting point than the longer fatty acids. Short-chain fatty acids also have fewer calories than longer ones, and are quickly absorbed from the digestive tract to be used for energy because they don't require breakdown by bile, so they are less likely to cause weight gain. Examples are propanoic acid, butyric acid, and caproic acid.

Medium-chain fatty acids. These have eight to twelve carbon atoms and, like short-chain fatty acids, are usually not deposited as fat because the body uses them quickly for cellular metabolism to produce energy. They are used in dietary formulas for people who need more fats for energy but cannot digest long-chain fatty acids. Athletes also use these fats for quick energy. Examples are caprylic acid, capric acid, and lauric acid. Tropical oils and butterfat contain medium-chain fatty acids.

Long-chain fatty acids. These fatty acids have fourteen to twenty-four carbon atoms. Some are EFAs that you need to take in from your diet directly, and some can be manufactured by your body from raw materials such as carbohydrates, protein, and other fatty acids provided by a good diet. Long-chain fatty acids have a higher melting point than our normal body temperature and are used to build cell membranes.

Saturated long-chain fatty acids are palmitic, stearic, myristic, and lauric acids. The body can make all of these except the EFA lauric acid. Coconut oil is 49 percent lauric acid and is known for its antimicrobial qualities. An interesting derivative of lauric acid, monolaurin, is present in palm kernel oil and tucum oil and is also strongly antimicrobial. Palmitic acid (16 carbons), found mainly in animal fats, and stearic acid (18 carbons) are the most common saturated fatty acids in foods. They can also be made in the body, and both can be converted to monounsaturated fatty acids if needed for some physiological function.

Monounsaturated long-chain fatty acids are palmitoleic acid and oleic acid, both of which can be made by the body. Oleic acid is also found in olive oil, pecans, almonds, cashews, and avocados.

Polyunsaturated long-chain fatty acids are EFAs, only obtained from the diet. They are best eaten in whole foods and in virgin cold-pressed oils. Keep these oils refrigerated and don't let them linger too long. If they cause a burning sensation in the back of your throat, they are rancid. Never use them for cooking. I cook with coconut oil, olive oil, or butter.

Examples of this type of fatty acid are the LNA and LA you've already read about. Another important polyunsaturated long-chain fatty acid is the omega-6 gamma linolenic acid (GLA), shown to help cardiovascular problems and is good for inflammatory conditions, weight loss, PMS, and skin and nail health. Primrose, borage, and black currant oils contain a good amount of GLA. You can find these in most health food stores.

Don't get GLA confused with CLA, which stands for conjugated linoleic acid. CLA is a polyunsaturated long-chain fatty acid found in meats and is therefore difficult to obtain on a vegetarian diet. Research biochemist Michael Pariza found that CLA has anti-carcinogenic properties, and recent research has shown that it helps to normalize fat deposition and prevent weight gain.

Lipids, Membranes, and Fat-Soluble Nutrients

Cellular membranes are primarily composed of special lipids, called phospholipids, and cholesterol. These lipids give flexibility and structure to the membranes and control what comes in and out of cells. You might recognize one phospholipid called phosphatidylcholine, also known as lecithin; it is found in egg yolks. Made up of palmitic and oleic acid, phosphatidylcholine increases the level of a neurotransmitter called acetylcholine, which carries neurological messages from brain cell to brain cell. Alzheimer's disease is characterized by a decrease in acetylcholine.

Another membrane phospholipid is phosphatidylserine, made up of stearic and oleic acid. Phosphatidylserine plays a role in giving brain cell membranes flexibility and structure. Researchers have used phosphatidyl-serine in the treatment of depression or impaired mental function in elderly patients including those with Alzheimer's. (On a related note, a myelin membrane consisting of 82 percent phospholipids wraps around nerve cells in the brain and central nervous system. A breakdown in this myelin sheath is found in some neurological diseases.)

Cholesterol is another important lipid that helps keep the structure and integrity of membranes intact. It is also a component of cellular receptors that bind with specific compounds so the cells can absorb them. Cholesterol is also needed for the skin cells' manufacture of vitamin D (in the form of provitamin D_3) and for the glands' production of hormones such as testosterone, estrogen, cortisol, and several others.

A point of interest is that without enough fats, you can become deficient in the fat-soluble vitamins A, D, E, and K. Fats help transport these and various other nutrients throughout the body. Deficiencies in fat-soluble nutrients have resulted from low-fat diets such as Pritikin's. Phytochemicals including lycopene, zeaxanthin, lutein, and carotenoids are fat-soluble antioxidants. Lutein and zeaxanthin have been proven to prevent macular degeneration, and research has shown that men with lycopene deficiency have a greater risk of developing prostate cancer.

Other fat-soluble nutrients include alpha lipoic acid, co-enzyme Q10, and carnitine. The body's utilization of all of these depends upon the presence of the proper amount and types of fatty acids. One nutrient always depends on one or more other nutrients to function properly—another plus for eating whole foods, which combine synergistic nutrients.

Omega Fatty Acids and Oxygen

Achieving peak oxygen absorption for your trillions of cells is a main goal for improved health, particularly because this greatly minimizes your susceptibility to cancer. The key to inhibiting the development of cancer is to maximize cells' oxidative metabolism—that is, raise their oxygen content. The cell membrane plays a crucial part in this endeavor. And what plays a crucial part in the cell membrane? EFAs. Every cell membrane is half protein and half fat. A portion of the membrane's fat is relatively non-reactive saturated fats, which absorb little oxygen. The other portion is unsaturated or polyunsaturated fats, which help the cell absorb oxygen. The saturated fats protect the unsaturated ones from lipid peroxidation by free radicals.

As long ago as 1910, Dr. Otto Warburg showed that if there is a 35 percent decrease in oxygen in the tissues, cancer can develop. Medical journals in 1996–1997 again reported the connection between decreased oxygen and increased cancer, describing it as "tumor hypoxia," or not having enough oxygen in the cells. *(Brizel DM, et al. Tissue oxygenation predicts for the likelihood of distant metastases in human soft tissue sarcoma. Cancer Res 1996 56:941-943; Brizel DM, et al. Tumor hypoxia adversely affects the prognosis of carcinoma of the head and neck. Int J Radiat Oncol Biol Phys 1997 38:285-290.)*

Here is where the EFAs play a role, as they are highly oxygen-absorbing fats—essentially, they act as magnets that grab oxygen from the bloodstream and transfer it into the cells. If you don't have enough of the right EFAs in your bloodstream, you are starving your cells of oxygen, which makes you more susceptible to cancer. Not only are the right EFAs important, but the ratio of one type to another matters as well.

Exercise is always a good way to increase oxygen in the body, but EFAs still must be present to transfer that oxygen into the cells. Having less of these fatty acids in the membranes means having less oxygen reaching the mitochondria, where respiration and energy production take place. Think about this in terms of being an athlete, or in terms of fatigue. We wonder why we are tired or don't recover from our exercise programs—perhaps it is because we aren't eating the right types and proportions of EFAs.

In 1929, researchers George and Mildred Burr reported a significant result of excluding fats from the diet, showing again that a lack of proper fats leads to low oxygen in the body, which can lead to cancer. *(Burr G, Burr M. A new deficiency disease produced by the rigid exclusion of fat from the diet. Biol Chem 1929 82:345-367.)* This finding coincided perfectly with Dr. Warburg's work—why wasn't it brought to the public's attention? Remember Dr. Warburg's statement, "The prime cause of cancer is insufficient oxygen to the cells." With an insufficient amount of EFAs, oxygen cannot be absorbed through the cellular membrane into the cell.

Cancer may have secondary causes, but the prime cause is a lack of oxygen. Respiration of oxygen is normal in a healthy cell. Cancer cells, however, manufacture their energy differently, by a fermentation process. Oxygen is relegated to a lower importance in cancer cells than in normal cells, because cancer cells especially love sugar. The fuel of fermentation is sugar. Fermentation leads to acidosis and promotes Candida overgrowth. You can see how the problem brings on a chain reaction of other diseases.

In a cancerous body, oxygen respiration is lowered and fermentation is increased, along with high levels of lactic acid. You can now see some of the mistakes athletes make. Not only do they produce large amounts of lactic acid, but a high-carbohydrate/high-sugar diet with EFA insufficiency and imbalanced ratios can lead to impaired athletic performance as well as rapid aging. Your cells produce more energy from normal respiration in the presence of omega fatty acids. For example, your liver and kidneys obtain 100 times more energy from respiration than from fermentation.

As you recall, EFAs must be supplied daily from food or supplements because your body cannot manufacture them. Organic seeds (such as sunflower, flax, and pumpkin) and nuts (such as almonds, walnuts, and cashews) are good sources, along with organic lean meats. Fish is not always the best source of EFAs because fish oils—in doing their job for the fish—rapidly absorb oxygen from the air and then spoil from oxidation.

There are two "parent" oils: the omega-3 LNA and the omega-6 LA. There are also "derivative" oils (derived from parent oils), which are used for supplements and claimed to be as good as the parent oil. For example, omega-3 derivatives are DHA and EPA; popular omega-6 derivatives are the previously mentioned CLA and GLA. Nothing is better than "the real thing," and in this case, the parent oils are the best. Medical research has shown that the body directly uses greater quantities of parent EFAs than their derivatives, up to twenty times more. It's not that supplements or derivatives are bad, but why not at least combine them with the real food?

The parent EFAs are normally converted into derivative components within the body (and also in the manufacture of some supplements). Some people's bodies, however, may not be able to make these nutritional conversions because of age or some metabolic problem. The answer is to correct the metabolic problem if possible, or at least combine the parent oils with derivatives, and use digestive enzymes to aid digestion.

Another problem is the over-processing of many commercially produced foods, as the processing changes their omega ratios, destroys parent oils, and loads them with cancer-causing trans fats that take longer to spoil because they have little oxygen-absorbing capacity. In the interests of long shelf-life, manufacturers of processed foods use ingredients and processes that destroy EFAs. Margarine, for instance, can be left out for years because of a process called hydrogenation (described later in this chapter)—however, hydrogenation creates trans fatty acids, which are toxic and associated with skin cancer.

Omega-3s and omega-6s should be eaten in a 1:1 ratio instead of the 1:20 ratio that is so common in the American diet and contributes to inflammation in your body. Unfortunately, the meat and milk of animals that are fed pesticide-impregnated foods and shot up with various hormones have imbalanced omega ratios. Feeding cattle grains and not grass changes the ratio drastically, up to 15:1 in favor of omega-6, compared to grass-fed cattle, which is about 1:1 to 3:1. Chicken and eggs from farm-raised hens who feed from a natural turf have a healthy 1:1 ratio of omega-6 to omega-3, whereas chicken and eggs from corn-fed, battery-raised hens have a 19:1 ratio of omega-6 to omega-3.

Unfortunately, most polyunsaturated vegetable oils contain only a little omega-3 and a lot of omega-6. Omega-3s are necessary for cellular oxidation and other important functions in every cell. Too much omega-6 can disrupt the cells' normal production of prostaglandins, which are hormone-like substances that generally act quickly and then vanish. Prostaglandins serve many yin-yang functions: for example, some are vasodilators that improve circulation, others are vasoconstrictors that raise blood pressure; some decrease inflammation, some increase inflammation; some increase pain, others decrease it; some cause blood platelet aggregation, some prevent it. By disturbing the proper balance of cellular oxidation and prostaglandin production, vegetable oils with excessive omega-6 can lead to digestive and immune disturbances.

Too much omega-3, however, can also be a bad thing. The problem with eating too much fish and taking concentrated fish oils as a source of omega EFAs is that they contain far too many omega-3s and thereby cause an imbalance between omega-3s and omega-6s. *(USDA Database: www.nal.usda.gov/fnic/foodcomp/search)* Dr. Dean Ornish also warns about fish oil, explaining that his colleague Dr. Alexander Leaf, though a proponent of omega-3s, found that his patients with congestive heart failure and recurrent angina got worse when taking fish oil: "For these people, it may kill them." *(www.newsweek.com/id/137192)* A review in the *British Medical Journal* found that the benefits of omega-3 consumption were mixed. *(Hooper L, et al. Risks and benefits of omega 3 fats for mortality, cardiovascular disease, and cancer: systematic review. BMJ 2006 332:752-760.)* It is important to realize that genetic ancestry, too, can affect the body's ability to utilize particular nutrients and food types.

Where Can We Get Our Omega Fatty Acids?

It's best to use virgin, cold-pressed oils. Make sure they are in dark bottles instead of aluminum containers (you already know the story on aluminum toxicity). It's estimated that we need 2–3 tablespoons daily of healthful oils.

EFA omega-3s can be found in walnut, flaxseed, soybean, and canola oil; the latter two, however, are not recommended. The omega-3s DHA and EPA can be made by the body, but people are often deficient in them anyway. Although fish oil has long been considered a good source of DHA and EPA, mercury poisoning from fish is a concern. If you decide to take fish oil, ask the manufacturer for a Technical Sheet to see the product's mercury level, and get your own mercury level checked every two years, as I do—mercury toxicity is not fun.

EFA omega-6s can be obtained from these oils: sunflower, evening primrose, corn, borage, flaxseed, and olive. As you can see, flaxseed oil has both omega-3 and omega-6 fatty acids. You can also use freshly ground flaxseed daily; I like to mix it into my smoothies. Some people put it on their cereal (however, I suggest avoiding grains, or at least keeping them to a minimum). As noted earlier, the omega-6 GLA is also found in borage oil, black currant oil, and evening primrose oil.

If you need supplemental EFAs, ProEFA from Nordic Naturals (800-662-2544) is an excellent product. Moss Nutrition offers a good omega-3 oil (have your licensed healthcare practitioner call 800-851-5444).

Tropical Oils Are Not the Enemy

Because of the bad press saturated fat has received over the years, tropical oils with a high content of saturated fat have been avoided or ignored. But these oils and fats do not contribute to heart disease unless they are hydrogenated (which would make any fat toxic). Coconut, palm, and palm kernel oils have long been used by cultures that have less cardiovascular disease than we do. Our understanding is finally catching up with what traditional cultures have known all along: that these tropical oils are, in fact, healthy. What has been shown recently is that the polyunsaturated, refined vegetable oils are the real culprits in disease. So I want to clear the air about a few fats and oils that have received a bad rap; I'm speaking of the tropical oils, especially coconut oil.

Coconut oil. Coconut oil contains the fatty acid lauric acid, which is an important constituent in infant formulas because it is also found in mother's milk. Coconut oil is also a good source of medium-chain fatty acids, described earlier in this chapter: its medium-chain fatty acids are 75 percent caprylic and 25 percent capric. The rest of coconut oil's fatty acids are 49 percent lauric, 8 percent palmitic, 2 percent stearic, 6 percent oleic, and 2 percent linolenic. What a tremendous food!

Coconut oil has been shown to withstand a wide heat range, which makes it good for cooking and frying. Make sure to buy extra-virgin coconut oil. It supports the thyroid, improves ratios of HDL and LDL cholesterol, and exhibits antibacterial, antiviral, and antifungal properties. I have used it with my clients for all types of intestinal inflammatory conditions such as irritable bowel syndrome and colitis, and for Candida overgrowth. (See Bruce Fife's book *The Healing Miracles of Coconut Oil*, published by Healthwise.)

Palm oil and palm kernel oil. Palm oil, made from the fresh fruit of the oil palm, is one of the most edible oils in the world. It contains 39 percent oleic, 45 percent palmitic, 9 percent linoleic, and 5 percent stearic acid, as well as some lauric acid—plus high levels of beta-carotene and other carotenoids. Palm kernel oil, on the other hand, is extracted from the nut of the palm fruit. It usually contains 50 percent lauric, 16 percent myristic, 8 percent palmitic, 14 percent oleic, and 2 percent linoleic acid.

Palm oil and palm kernel oil both contain the strong antioxidant vitamin E and its related tocotrienols. Vitamin E contains eight naturally occurring isomers, which are basically the same chemical compounds but have different configurations. Standard vitamin E, for example, has alpha, beta, gamma, and delta isomers called tocopherols. Other forms of vitamin E are called alpha, beta, gamma, and delta tocotrienols, which have been shown to be 40–60 percent more potent as antioxidants than standard vitamin E alone.

I suggest taking vitamin E and its tocotrienols together. Palm oil has 256 milligrams per kilogram of tocopherols and tocotrienols, compared to palm kernel oil's 13 milligrams. Because of their saturated fats, both palm and palm kernel oil are very stable. They can be kept at room temperature for months and are excellent for baking and frying at low temperatures.

Olive oil. Olive oil is the main vegetable oil used in Greece, Spain, and Italy. The very first cold pressing of the olives yields oil that is called virgin cold-pressed and is the most nutritious (as long as it is kept in dark bottles). Its fatty acid composition is 14 percent palmitic, 71 percent oleic, 10 percent linoleic, and 1 percent LNA. Because of its high content of monounsaturated long-chain oleic acid, olive oil is very stable, but it has a tendency to be deposited in the body's fat cells, unlike oils that have short or medium-chain fatty acids.

Flaxseed oil. Flaxseed oil, a "king among oils," has been used in clinical situations for LNA deficiency. Its omega-3s provide a natural remedy for major degenerative conditions such as cancer, cardiovascular disease, diabetes, multiple sclerosis (MS), arthritis, and other inflammatory diseases. Taking flaxseed oil daily helps reduce the body's accumulation of trans fats and has also been shown to lower blood pressure. Flaxseed oil is 9 percent saturated fatty acids, 18 percent oleic acid, 16 percent omega-6, and 57 percent omega-3. Because of its high omega-3 content, it helps correct omega-3 and omega-6 imbalances—remember, we consume too many omega-6 fatty acids (such as LA) from polyunsaturated vegetable oils. Never heat flaxseed oil.

Less-favored oils. The omega-6 polyunsaturated LA constitutes 59 percent of the fat in corn oil, 68 percent in sunflower seed oil, and a whopping 78 percent in safflower oil. Omega-6s can be troublesome if consumed in excess. These oils should only be ingested sparingly, if at all. They go rancid quickly and should not be used for cooking.

Canola oil, also called rape-seed oil, should not be consumed by humans. It contains a long-chain fatty acid called erucic acid, which has been shown to be toxic and is associated with heart disease. This oil also goes rancid easily and forms molds that you definitely want to avoid.

Peanut oil is 42 percent oleic acid, 15 percent saturated fat, but 34 percent linoleic acid. Like olive oil, it is stable and therefore good for cooking, but as with most oils high in omega-6s, it should only be used in small amounts. Also beware of a potential toxic fungus called aflatoxin that is sometimes associated with peanut products; choose organic peanut oil to be safe, as organic farming and harvesting make it less likely to be contaminated with aflatoxin.

Sesame oil is 41 percent oleic, 43 percent linoleic, and 10 percent palmitic acid. Like olive oil, its oleic acid makes it good for cooking, but keep its use at a minimum because of the high omega-6 content.

What we originally thought was harmful, saturated tropical oil, is what we actually do want to help reduce weight and fight infection. Keep your use of vegetable oils at a minimum because of their polyunsaturated omega-6 fats. They go rancid quickly, and their long-chain fatty acids tend to put on weight. Increase your omega-3s by eating fish (but watch for mercury) and flaxseeds or flaxseed oil.

Hydrogenation and Trans Fats

As mentioned earlier, hydrogenated fats are used in the food-processing industry because they are inexpensive and provide various products with shelf-life stability—but at the expense of our health and the loss of the food's nutritional value. Hydrogenation drastically changes natural oils by combining them with hydrogen gas at temperatures of 240–410°F. Metals such as nickel, platinum, copper, and aluminum are also involved. All double bonds in the oils become saturated with hydrogen, leaving no polyunsaturated oil in its natural state, but rather an unnatural, toxic, trans fat contaminated by heavy metals—those facts, of course, are not publicly advertised.

Hydrogenation and its incomplete version, partial hydrogenation, both create large quantities of trans fatty acids (TFAs). Products such as margarine, the latest generation of butter substitutes, vegetable shortening, and some vegetable oils are partially hydrogenated. Margarine and shortening contain about 20 percent TFAs.

No doubt you've heard about these unhealthy trans fats. Eating them upsets your natural fatty acid metabolism at the cellular level and crowds out the EFAs that you need. The body cannot use hydrogenated or partially hydrogenated fats and oils in the same way it uses natural fats and oils, because their original structure has been altered. Specifically, a slight deviation in the rotation of the oil molecule around a double bond, which occurs during processing, changes the molecule from cis to trans configuration; see the diagram below.

Molecular structure of cis fatty acid versus trans fatty acid

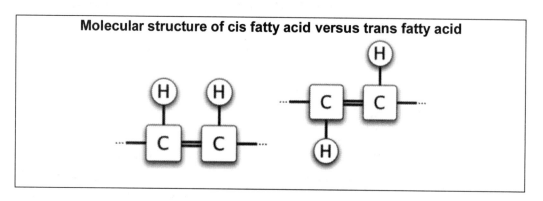

TFAs are produced by subjecting any form of fat to high temperatures, as occurs during full or partial hydrogenation and also some types of cooking such as frying. When the fat is heated to 160°C or higher, the hydrogen atoms that were in a cis configuration on the same side of the fatty acid molecule switch to the opposite side. This trans configuration is more stable than the cis configuration, but because it is no longer a natural fatty acid, it no longer fits properly into cellular membranes and enzymes. It tends to change the ability of the cell to absorb certain nutrients and also allows the entry of destructive substances. As a result, the cell's protective barrier is systematically destroyed.

TFAs are very difficult for the body to break down. They cause blood cells to stick together, leading to plaque deposits in the liver and arteries that increase the risk of strokes and heart attacks. Eating TFAs can increase your cholesterol levels by 15 percent and triglycerides by 45 percent, in addition to decreasing beneficial HDL. By interfering with the enzyme systems that metabolize natural fatty acids, TFAs can cause fatty acid deficiencies. TFAs have also been shown to interfere with liver function and other bodily detoxification systems.

Don't eat hydrogenated or partially hydrogenated fats if you can possibly avoid it. Ninety-five percent of dietary TFAs come from hydrogenated oils, margarine, and shortenings; others come from partially hydrogenated oils. These substances are found in many, many foods—so it is important to read labels, because hydrogenated and partially hydrogenated fats are listed by name, and you can avoid eating them.

Using Fats to Your Advantage

Knowing which fats are antifungal, antiviral, and antibacterial is a great asset when working with specific diseases. Good fats are also required for healing injuries such as bruises, strains, and sprains, for the oxygenation of tissues, for the oxidation that produces energy within cells, and for numerous other functions in a healthy body. Bad fats, especially trans fats, can slow down all these processes and hinder your body's performance on many levels.

For recovery from any disease and from exercise, avoid processed oils, fried and rancid fats and oils, and hydrogenated or partially hydrogenated oils. These substances injure cell membranes, inhibit cellular respiration (which is necessary for the oxidation of food), and interfere with circulation and liver functions. They can also interfere with normal digestive functions, irritate the bowels, and cause allergic reactions.

As you've read in earlier chapters, what sets up the conditions for pleomorphism and the spread of bacteria and fungus is an acidic terrain. Fat that is processed, overcooked, or in a trans configuration can produce an acidic terrain by interfering with cells' oxygen uptake and literally

236236

236   *ProMetabolics Part Three: Cleansing and Optimizing*

blocking the elimination of cellular acid wastes. It is impossible to have a healthy cellular environment with unnatural fatty acids causing these conditions. Unnatural fats produce an acidic and congested terrain, which can lead to the development of almost any degenerative disease you can think of.

In summary, it's a good idea to increase your intake of EFAs—keeping the omega-6 to omega-3 ratio 1:1, no more than 3:1—in combination with eating a low-carb, low-sugar diet that's high in green foods, and getting plenty of exercise. Here's a helpful bottom line:

- Eat fish; don't take large amounts of fish oils, if any at all. (All fish contain some mercury.)
- Use seed and nut oils, as well as some extra-virgin olive oil, all of them organic and cold-pressed.
- Read Brian Scott Peskin's book *The Hidden Story of Cancer* (published by Pinnacle Press).
- Stay off sugar.
- Watch your pH and monitor your foods as described in this book so you won't become too acidic.
- Keep your omega-6 to omega-3 ratio 1:1 (equal parts). When you're eating natural foods and especially if most of your foods are organic, an imbalance in fatty acid intake is highly unlikely.
- Remember, the healthiest people in the world know nothing of these things. They have no research and probably can't read. So just keep it natural!

ENZYMES AND HEALTH

One of the most important components of good health is digestion. In addition to bringing necessary nutrients into the body, proper digestion and a healthy digestive tract serve as our first line of defense against disease. Monitoring pH and temperature is an asset in improving digestion because all enzymes—whether in the blood, digestive tract, or other organs—work best in specific temperature and pH conditions. If your digestive enzymes are not functioning properly because your pH has been disturbed, the nutrients contained within your foods are not liberated for absorption. Furthermore, undigested foods often cause fermentation and gas, acidifying the whole digestive tract—and that process can lead to leaky bowel syndrome, allergies, fibromyalgia, acid reflux, and other inflammatory diseases.

We hear so much about vitamins, minerals, proteins, fats, and carbohydrates, but we seldom hear about the body's real labor force: enzymes. As stated in a 1966 medical report, "Each of us, as with all living organisms, could be regarded as an orderly, integrated succession of enzyme reactions." Enzymes are needed for every chemical action and reaction in the body. Metabolic enzymes run your organs, tissues, and cells. Nutrients and hormones can't do their work unless particular enzymes are present. And if your enzymes aren't doing their jobs, it is difficult if not impossible to balance your terrain—that's why I suggest using supplemental enzymes in so many situations. In turn, keeping your terrain in balance supports proper enzyme activity and function.

Throughout my years of experience as a health practitioner, author, and researcher, I came to understand that no singular formula, food, or health product is a "cure-all." Nevertheless, I felt that there had to be something that every person could use as a regular health supplement, or as a foundation and adjunct to both medical and non-medical therapies.

Eventually, I realized that supplemental digestive enzymes were what I'd been searching for. If you are interested in longevity, vitality, superior health, and overcoming sickness, or if you're having trouble losing weight, or if you've taken vitamins and minerals for years but haven't benefited as much as you hoped to, this chapter should be of special interest to you.

What Are Enzymes, and What Do They Do in the Body?

It is often said that enzymes are protein molecules, but that description is inadequate. Let me clarify this with the analogy of a light bulb, which can only light up when you put an electric current through it. We can say that the light bulb has a dual nature: a physical structure, and a non-physical force that is expressed through it. So think of an enzyme's structure, a protein molecule, as the carrier of the enzyme's invisible activity or energy factor, much like the bulb is the carrier for the current.

Experiments described as far back as 1933 showed that the activity of such a protein molecule can even be transferred to another, leaving the original molecule devoid of its original activity. An intact and "animated" enzyme can do its specific job such as digesting food, building tissues, or aiding detoxification. However, under certain circumstances such as high temperature or altered pH, the enzyme can be destroyed in the sense that it can no longer perform its function—although the molecule is still physically present, the energy that once animated it is no longer present.

Enzymes do a tremendous amount of work. They are involved in every process of the body, and life could not exist without them. Start with digestion: Enzymes break your food down into particles small enough to pass through the pores of the intestinal wall. Enzymes in the bloodstream incorporate those nutrients into your muscles, nerves, blood, and glands.

Furthermore, all cellular activities are initiated by enzymes. Enzymes assist in storing sugar in the liver and muscles and storing fat in adipose tissue. They aid in the elimination of carbon dioxide from the lungs and in the formation of urea to be excreted as urine. Enzymes break down toxins so the body can expel them without damaging the eliminative organs. An enzyme helps attach iron to red blood cells. Sperm carries enzymes that dissolve the membrane of the egg. An enzyme called streptokinase is used in medicine to dissolve blood clots. And these are only a few examples of enzyme involvement in your everyday bodily functions.

The number of different enzymes in the body is overwhelming, and yet each one has a particular job to do—they are very "intelligent" when it comes to their activity and functions. This is called enzyme specificity: for example, a protein-digesting enzyme will not act on a fat, and a fat-digesting enzyme will not act on a starch. Enzymes act upon a given substance, called a substrate, and change the substrate into another substance with a different identity, but the enzymes remain unchanged themselves. Each enzyme is believed to fit into a specific geometrical design, as shown on the following page.

How An Enzyme Works

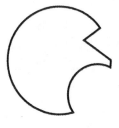
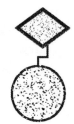

Enzyme Before Working   **Molecule Complete**

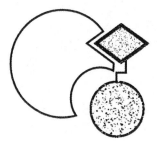

Enzyme While Working

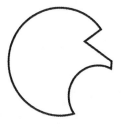
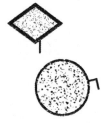

Enzyme After Working   **Molecule Split Apart**

From *The Chemicals of Life* by Isaac Asimov
Illustrated by John Bradford, New American Library, 1954

Enzymes are a component of all living matter. Since 1968, 1,300 enzymes have been identified in the human body. There are three major classes: metabolic enzymes (enzymes that work in blood, tissues, and organs), food enzymes from raw food, and digestive enzymes. Our organs are run by metabolic enzymes, which build tissues out of food substances and also have numerous other duties. One authority found ninety-eight different enzymes working in the arteries alone. A shortage of metabolic enzymes may cause serious health problems.

The names of most enzymes, though not all, end in "-ase," and in most cases, the name of the enzyme (or the group it belongs to) also reveals its function. This is illustrated by the four categories of digestive enzymes: lipases, which break down fat; proteases, which break down protein; cellulases, which break down cellulose; and amylases, which break down starch. Each category contains a number of specific enzymes. Among the proteases, for instance, are the proteolytic enzymes trypsin and pepsin. (The word "proteolytic" is just the singular form of the word "protease.")

The names are not important unless you are going to make enzymes a topic of study. What is important is to understand the sources of enzymes and how to get more enzymes into your body. The more enzyme-deficient you become, the faster you age. The more you build up your enzyme reserve, the healthier you will be.

Where Do We Get Our Enzymes?

We usually think of enzymes as involved only in digesting our food—we seldom consider that enzymes are involved in every metabolic process, every organ and system, and our ability to see, think, and breathe. Any degree of depletion of the enzymes that function in any of these areas can be detrimental. Much literature has tried to establish toxicity and genetics as predisposing factors in disease, but we must realize that a lack of enzymes can predispose the body to disease as well.

You lose enzymes daily through your sweat, urine, feces, and all digestive fluids including saliva and intestinal secretions. It is very important to preserve and replenish your enzyme levels at all cost. There are two ways to do this: by eating raw food and by taking enzyme supplements.

If you had two seeds and boiled one of them, which of the two would grow when placed in soil? There is no question that the unboiled seed would sprout, and that's because its enzymes would still be intact. Similarly, the difference between "live" (raw) and "dead" (cooked) food is enzymatic activity. All foods provided by nature, when in their raw state, contain an abundance of enzymes, which are there to aid in the food's digestion so the body is not forced to produce all the enzymes needed for all that work. However, one general characteristic of enzymes is an inability to withstand very hot temperatures—such as those in cooking.

At 129°F, all enzymes are destroyed. This happens quite rapidly when live food substances come in contact with heated water. According to enzyme therapy pioneer Dr. Edward Howell, "Enzymes are more or less completely destroyed when heated in water in the temperature range between 48 degrees to 65 degrees Centigrade. Long heating at 48 degrees Centigrade or short heating at 65 degrees Centigrade kills enzymes. Heating at 60 to 80 degrees Centigrade for one-half hour completely kills any enzymes."

Consequently, enzymes are completely destroyed in all foods that have been canned, pasteurized, baked, boiled, broiled, roasted, stewed, or fried. Take a moment to consider how many foods that encompasses. Processing, cooking, and more recently microwaving dramatically and detrimentally change the food you eat. These actions render your foods enzyme-deficient, causing imbalances in your organs and acting as a predisposing factor in disease.

Animals in the wild consume large amounts of enzymes that are naturally present in their raw food diets. This aids in digestion and takes much of the burden off organs such as the pancreas, liver, and spleen. Without the help of those raw foods, the animals would have to produce large amounts of digestive enzymes, causing unwarranted stress on those organs and other tissues and decreasing their longevity.

We're born with an enzyme reserve, but this is subsequently decreased over years of eating an enzyme-deficient diet. Because we eat most of our food cooked, our digestive system has to produce all of the enzymes to digest it. To meet that demand, the body must draw metabolic enzymes and precursors for making digestive enzymes from all of its organs and tissues, causing a metabolic deficit. If you take in more enzymes from your diet and other sources, however, your enzyme reserve would not be depleted so rapidly, and your metabolic enzymes would remain more evenly distributed throughout your body. This is one of the most health-promoting measures that you can implement in your daily lifestyle.

The pancreas, which as you know is of primary importance to the digestive system, secretes lipase, amylase, and protease. Even when the pancreas is experimentally removed in animals, however, a certain enzyme level is still maintained in the body. It would be too much to expect an organ weighing just a few ounces (the average pancreas weighs only 85 grams) to supply, single-handedly, the enormous amount of enzymes needed to digest all your food day after day, year after year. It turns out that the pancreas also receives enzymes that have been manufactured elsewhere in the body. Enzymes have been found in all of our organs and tissues. White blood cells, for example, contain an even greater variety of enzymes than the pancreas.

A point of paramount importance is that a percentage of any enzymes taken orally or eaten in raw foods can be absorbed through the intestinal wall and utilized in the body's metabolic processes, counteracting enzyme depletion. In one study, Dr. A.W. Oelgoetz gave a pancreatic extract containing amylase to patients with low blood amylase, and their amylase levels normalized within one hour and remained normal for days. *(Oelgoetz AW, et al. The treatment of food allergy and indigestion of pancreatic origin with pancreatic enzymes. Am J Dig Dis Nutr 1935 2:422-426.)*

This finding has a very significant connection to some other substances absorbed through the intestines. As you learned earlier in this book, the passage of yeast cells and undigested food constituents such as proteins from the digestive tract into the bloodstream can cause allergies, skin diseases, and other illnesses. The bloodstream, however, provides the ideal environment for enzymes to help break down such undigested materials. Dr. Oelgoetz showed that when patients with allergies and low blood enzyme levels were given supplemental pancreatic enzymes, their levels normalized and their allergies subsided. Functional digestive disturbances and hyperacidity have been relieved the same way, as have a variety of skin diseases caused by incompletely digested food materials. Similarly, Drs. Max Wolf and Karl Ransberger have administered proteolytic enzymes for years to treat inflammation and sports injuries (see their book *Enzyme Therapy*, from Vantage Press).

Raw Foods, Enzymes, and Predigestion

It is certainly possible to live for many years on a cooked food diet, but eventually this causes cellular enzyme exhaustion, laying the foundation for a weak immune system and ultimately for disease. As described by Dr. Howell, "Researchers show that cooked food with the fiber broken down passes through the digestive system more slowly than raw foods. Partially it ferments, rots, and putrefies, throwing back into the body toxins, gas, and causing heartburn and degenerative diseases."

A human being is not maintained by the food that is taken in but rather by the portion that is actually digested. Every food must be broken down by enzymes into simpler building blocks. As has been noted, enzymes may be exogenous (from outside of the body) or endogenous (from within the body). The more exogenous enzymes you get from raw foods or from supplements, the less you need to borrow from your metabolic processes and supply from your organs.

As it turns out, the particular enzymes contained in a given raw food actually aid in the digestion of that same food once it is chewed. They break down 5–40 percent of the raw food without the help of the body's endogenous enzymes. Significant energy and enzymes are conserved when the body does not have to supply 100 percent of the enzymes necessary for digestion. Knowing how to use raw foods and supplemental enzymes in the diet is tremendously advantageous. Well-known naturalists such as Arnold Ehret, Ann Wigmore, George J. Drews, and Viktoras Kulvinskas have demonstrated the healing effects of raw foods.

This activity of exogenous food enzymes takes place primarily in the upper part of the stomach. *Gray's Anatomy* cites the authority Walter B. Cannon, who demonstrated that the human stomach "consists of two parts physiologically distinct... The cardiac portion of the stomach is a food reservoir in which salivary digestion continues; the pyloric portion is the seat of active gastric digestion. There are no peristaltic waves in the cardiac portion." (*Gray's Anatomy, 39th ed. Elsevier Churchill Livingstone, New York, NY, 2004.*) Anatomically speaking, the cardiac and fundic portions of the stomach are the enzyme-stomach, where raw foods are predigested by their own enzymes.

Major Regions Of The Stomach

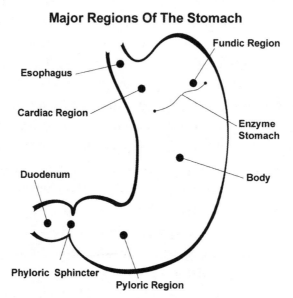

Illustration by Eric Lindley

Predigestion by exogenous enzymes is widespread in nature, and the enzyme-stomach is not unique to humans. Cattle and sheep have no salivary enzymes but have four stomachs, only one of which secretes endogenous enzymes; the other stomachs let the food's enzymes do the predigesting. Predigestion also occurs in one of the three stomachs of dolphins and whales. As many as thirty-two seals were once found in one whale's enzyme-stomach; with no enzymes secreted into this stomach by the whale, how could all that food get broken down enough to pass through a small opening into the next stomach? The enzymes in the flesh of the eaten animal itself seem to be the only answer.

In your enzyme-stomach, where no acid secretion or peristalsis takes place, supplemental enzymes and food enzymes can predigest a good percentage of your food for one-half to one hour after it is eaten and before it reaches your small intestine. The importance of this process cannot be overestimated. The pancreas secretes its digestive enzymes into the duodenum (the first part of the small intestine); if your food has not been properly predigested, your pancreas is put under tremendous stress to produce a lot of digestive enzymes and may need to draw enzymes from elsewhere to get the job done.

Your enzyme reserve has much more useful (and very taxing) work to do aside from providing digestive enzymes to break down your food. Predigestion greatly relieves the body's digestive burden, because the draw on its metabolic enzymes is minimized. This principle is called the adaptive secretion of digestive enzymes: the more digestion is accomplished in the stomach by food enzymes or supplemental enzymes, the more enzymes can be conserved for metabolic processes such as repairing tissues and organs. And the more digestion takes place before food reaches your small intestine, the better it is for your pancreas and intestines as well as for your whole body's integrity, strength, and immunity.

A number of experiments have demonstrated the digestive assistance of enzymes in raw foods. And although it was once believed that all food enzymes were destroyed in the stomach, this assumption has been overturned. Some food enzymes not only work in the stomach, but continue their activity in the small intestine. In one study, supplemental amylase was found to digest starch in the stomach, pass uninjured into the small intestine, and continue digestion there. Dr. Steven Boas demonstrated that enzymes in bananas were inactivated in the stomach but then reactivated in the intestines to aid in the bananas' digestion. Similarly, Russian researcher Dr. Matveev demonstrated that enzymes from carrot juice (oxidase and catalase) were inactivated in the stomach's acidity and then reactivated in the alkalinity of the small intestine.

If food is overcooked and its inherent enzymes destroyed, the only enzymes that get mixed with the food in the enzyme stomach are those in saliva. Some starch may be digested thanks to salivary amylase, but otherwise, practically no digestion occurs during the food's allotted time in the enzyme stomach. Protein is acted upon by the stomach's pepsin, but mostly in the lower part of the stomach. Fat remains practically untouched until it moves into the small intestine, where it can be acted on by pancreatic lipase.

As a result, cooked foods, especially those high in protein, can begin putrefying in the intestines. The byproducts of putrefaction are toxins that are absorbed into the bloodstream and deposited in tissues elsewhere. So you can see how valuable enzymes are in keeping the blood clear of such poisons; it's been estimated that 80 percent of diseases are caused by the body's absorption of improperly digested foods and their byproducts.

Enzymes, Disease, and Longevity

Studying the enzyme content in the blood, urine, and digestive fluids of the human population yields very telling data. It has been shown that young adults have a high level of enzyme reserve in their tissues, whereas in older adults the enzyme reserve is much lower. As noted, the average diet is predominantly heat-treated and therefore possesses only a fraction of its original (raw) enzyme content. When a young person eats cooked food, there is a greater outpouring of enzymes from the organs, tissues, and body fluids than in an older person. This is because years of eating a cooked food diet has depleted the older person's enzyme reserve.

An experiment at Chicago's Michael Reese Hospital with one group of participants aged twenty-one to thirty-one and another group aged sixty-nine to one hundred showed that the young group had thirty times more amylase in their saliva than the elderly group. *(Meyer J, Necheles H. Studies in old age. IV. The clinical significance of salivary, gastric, and pancreatic secretion in the aged. JAMA 1940 115:2050.)* This demonstrates why younger people can tolerate a diet full of white bread, starches, and predominantly cooked food. But as your enzyme reserve becomes depleted over the years, these same foods can cause problems such as constipation, blood diseases, ulcers, bloating, and arthritis. In older people whose enzyme reserve is lower, these foods are not properly digested and instead ferment in the digestive tract, producing toxins that are then absorbed into the bloodstream and deposited in the joints and soft tissues.

A chronic condition is a constant drag on the body's stored nutrients and other resources. In any chronic disease state, there is usually a low enzyme reserve. One study of 111 tuberculosis patients showed that 82 percent of them had lower enzyme levels than normal individuals, and as the disease worsened, enzyme levels decreased further. Dr. Leonid Volodin found that enzymes in the urine, blood, and intestines are usually decreased in diabetics; five of six diabetic patients also had reduced lipase and trypsin in their pancreatic secretions. Dr. D.M. Ottenstein found low blood amylase in patients with psoriasis, dermatitis, and pruritus. Another study showed that forty patients with liver disease (cirrhosis or hepatitis) or gall bladder inflammation (cholecystitis) had low blood amylase, and that when their amylase was increased, they experienced improvement in their specific disease as well as their general condition.

In acute disease, and sometimes at the start of chronic disease, the enzyme content in blood, tissues, urine, and feces is often found to be high. In such cases, the body's reserve is not yet depleted, which enables a larger outpouring of enzymes in the battle against disease; but as the disease progresses, the body's enzyme content is lowered. Strangely enough, although enzyme levels during chronic disease and during old age are similarly diminished, a low level in old age is typically seen as "normal," whereas a low level in chronic disease is seen as pathological.

The truth is that age is not so much a matter of how many years you have been alive, but rather of the integrity of your body's tissues. The metabolism of every cell in these tissues depends upon the enzymes that are present. There is a definite correlation between the amount of enzymes an individual possesses and the amount of energy he or she has. Furthermore, enzymes are a huge anti-aging factor, probably more important than any other. No doubt you've noticed that people age at considerably different rates—some fifty-year-olds look forty, others look sixty—and this has a lot to do with their enzyme levels.

As you age, your enzyme reserve slowly decreases. When enzyme levels become so low that metabolism suffers, death is the ultimate result. Any time metabolism is falsely hyped up by coffee or other stimulants, enzymes are used up in an output of false energy. Although you feel a sense of well-being, the end result is lower energy, a more rapid burnout of enzymes, and premature old age. At the University of Toronto, a team of scientists showed that the aging process runs in direct proportion to the body's catabolic rate—that is, the rate of wear and tear, or of tissue breakdown. This breakdown happens to be performed by enzymes, so the faster the breakdown, the more quickly the body's enzymes are used up.

Your enzyme reserve can be used up rapidly or it can be preserved. Taking enzyme supplements and eating raw foods are ways to add to your reserve and to boost your energy level as well. As Dr. Howell states, "Enzymes are a true yardstick of vitality. Enzymes offer an important means of calculating the vital energy of an organism. That which we call energy, vital force, nerve energy, and strength, may be synonymous with enzyme activity." When your enzyme level is lowered, your metabolism is lowered, and so is your energy level. Do not misunderstand—I am not saying that enzymes are the sole source of life. The message here is that there is a correlation among the enzyme levels in an organism's tissues, the youthfulness of those tissues, and the energy level of the organism.

Enzymes for Everybody

I cannot urge strongly enough that you preserve and replenish your body's enzyme reserve. To that end, the importance of eating raw food is undeniable. Taking supplemental digestive enzymes can also be tremendously helpful—on a regular basis, during detoxification diets, and when digestive problems present themselves. If you eat mostly cooked food, you should take supplemental enzymes. As you use the monitoring system, you will see that these enzymes are key to improving your digestion and balancing your internal terrain. Enzyme supplementation is also necessary in almost all acute or chronic health conditions. (For more information on enzymes, please see my book, *Food Enzymes: The Missing Link to Radiant Health*, from Hohm Press.)

When you buy any enzyme supplement, be sure that it does not contain animal-derived enzymes. Plant- or aspergillus-derived enzymes, however, are fine. Ideally, you want a product that contains all four types of digestive enzymes: amylase, protease, lipase, and cellulase. These are available at most health food stores as well as from online distributors such as Mountain States Health Products.

PART FOUR

ProMetabolics: Nutritional Strategies for Disease Prevention and Health Enhancement

DIGESTION AND DETOXIFICATION: EATING AND CLEANSING THE PROMETABOLIC WAY

This chapter describes how to eat according to your body's natural digestive and detoxification cycles. Central to this is the knowledge that your body cleanses itself while you're sleeping, eliminates wastes and toxins in the morning, and is then prepared to digest food during the day and early evening. Following the digestive and cleansing cycles of the body is one of the most important factors in health and healing.

These cycles are why, for example, you shouldn't eat within three hours before bedtime. If you do, you throw the body into digestion mode while you're trying to sleep. Why is that a bad thing? Because it means the body can't cleanse itself as it's supposed to; toxins build up in the intestines; reserves of buffering minerals are used up to neutralize toxins and balance the blood's pH; the normal cycle of hormone production and secretion is thrown off; and sleep is disrupted. And as if that weren't bad enough, all of those things make you age more rapidly.

The eating and cleansing cycle I'm talking about is nothing new, and your cells and hormonal cycles remember it well. Consider our early hunting and gathering ancestors, who exercised daily, went long periods of time without food, and kept lean. They did not sit in an office and gorge themselves with three huge meals a day when they weren't hungry. Their brains automatically reset their bodies' day and night cycles every day in response to light exposure—and so do ours. We no longer live our ancestors' lifestyle, but we still have their genes.

One of the fundamentals of prometabolic eating is, in fact, to eat like a hunter-gatherer. You'll feel energized and clear-minded as you naturally adapt to this way of eating—and you'll even find that it is cheaper and easier to eat this way. You will enable your body to work at peak efficiency by following its built-in hormonal, catabolic/anabolic, and enzyme cycles. And it's so much fun knowing that you're in control of your health.

Your Natural Metabolic Cycle

Strenuous body detoxification programs such as fasting and other therapeutic cleansing diets are outside the scope of this book. You should only undergo such programs with the supervision of a qualified healthcare practitioner. What I'm talking about in this chapter is how to eat and use supplements so your body is self-regulating according to its innate cleansing and digesting cycles. During these cycles, you can monitor and balance your pH using foods and suggested supplementation while you also observe what's happening with your endocrine glands.

The organ clock below illustrates how energy travels from one organ system to the next. This chart is more than 2,000 years old and is principally used by physicians of Chinese medicine. There is always energy in all organs and tissues, but during specific times of the day or night, certain organs have more energy traveling through them and become more active. This is your body's natural metabolic cycle.

Organ Clock

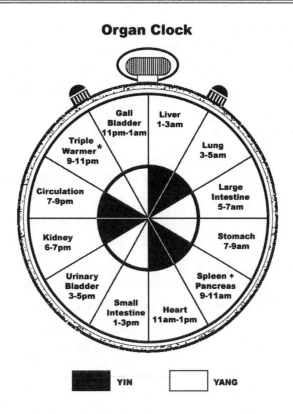

YIN   YANG

* Triple Warmer in Chinese medicine refers to the circulation of heat, including the thyroid and adrenal glands.

Look on the organ clock at the period between 7:00 a.m. and 11:00 a.m. This is a good time to eat, when more energy is in the stomach, spleen, and enzyme-secreting pancreas. Then throughout the rest of the day, the more active organs are those responsible for circulation, such as the heart, kidneys, and bladder.

In contrast, look at the organs that are more active from 11:00 p.m. to 7:00 a.m.: gall bladder, liver, lungs, and large intestine. During those sleeping hours, your body is detoxifying and preparing to eliminate wastes in the early morning. When you awaken, what is the first thing you do? Go to the bathroom. It's the natural thing to do.

It has been scientifically demonstrated that the body's physiology naturally coordinates with this energetic cycle. So don't disturb it! You can observe, control, and support this cycle by self-monitoring and by feeding your body what it needs, when it needs it. Again, this is not a dramatic cleansing diet; it's just supporting natural prometabolic cycles—especially the anti-aging detox cycle—for better health.

Building Up and Breaking Down: Anabolism and Catabolism

Don't fall for the theory that it's good to eat six small meals during the day. Not only will you drive yourself crazy, but if you're always eating, you're continually using up your enzyme reserve and digesting; you're accomplishing less body purification; and there's constantly food sitting in your intestines. This sets you up for intestinal fermentation, which leads to gas, digestive problems, and Candida overgrowth.

Your body's fundamental metabolic processes of anabolism and catabolism are significantly affected by when and what you eat. Anabolism is the building-up process in the body. During anabolism, amino acids are joined together to build and repair tissues. Protein is deposited in muscle tissue and fat in adipose tissue. Toxins from the bloodstream are deposited as well. Excess sugar, other carbohydrates, and fats are stored as triglycerides for later fuel.

An important reminder about "building up": you don't get fat by eating natural fats from such foods as avocadoes and soaked seeds and nuts—it's the cooked, processed, and high-carbohydrate foods that put the weight on. The worst offenders are excessive unnatural sugars and other high-carb foods such as processed grains, potatoes, cookies, corn products, and pasteurized juices. They turn to fat in the body; they create heavy mucus and congest your filtering organs; and they cause fatigue and raise blood sugar. Avoiding them will help prevent hypoglycemia.

Hypoglycemia is the result of a sudden rise in blood sugar, which causes your insulin level to spike, which in turn causes a sudden blood sugar drop or "crash."

Controlling insulin levels is the key to weight loss—which may be the greatest weight-related secret of all time. As mentioned, eating lots of sugar and processed high-carb foods leads to high insulin secretion and the conversion of your excess blood sugar into fat for storage. Furthermore, insulin inhibits fat breakdown, and you get fatter. Although an overly high insulin level is anabolic, you pay the price (in weight and other insulin-related problems) in the long run.

Catabolism is the other half of the metabolic cycle, the breaking-down process. During catabolism, the body breaks down various compounds: glycogen is broken into glucose, triglycerides into fatty acids, and protein into amino acids. These building blocks are then used for fuel and for building in anabolism. As you may have guessed, both the building-up and breaking-down processes must be supported with proper nutrients. Furthermore, optimal balance between catabolic and anabolic metabolism is impossible without a properly functioning endocrine system (pituitary, thyroid, adrenals, and ovaries/testes).

Detoxification works best when anabolism and catabolism are in balance. Your eliminatory organs must also be kept healthy and clear to keep up with the necessary elimination of wastes and toxins. Sweating and exercise are important for your natural cleansing processes as well.

Being aware of your body's metabolic cycle puts you in control. Using the monitoring system will tell you what you need to support your cycle. Monitor your terrain's pH, and if need be, monitor your thyroid, adrenal, and pituitary activity as well. If you see an imbalance, you can consult your ProMetabolics Terrain-Balancing Chart and eat and supplement accordingly. It feels so good to know that you're in control of your health.

The Key to ProMetabolic Eating

Why do I keep talking about how sugars, other high-carb foods, and overeating stimulate insulin secretion? Today we have an epidemic called Syndrome X, consisting of insulin resistance/hyperinsulinism, type II diabetes, hypoglycemia, insulin sensitivity, and other problems including high triglyceride levels. It is often accompanied by obesity as well. All of the health problems associated with Syndrome X are due to improper eating and not understanding the natural eating cycles of the body.

Furthermore, eating high-carb and cooked foods—and too much food—overworks the pancreas, which has to secrete huge amounts of enzymes to digest it all. You've learned how important it is to preserve your body's enzyme supply to counteract aging and keep your immune system healthy. Enzyme deficiency, old age, and chronic disease should be thought of as synonymous terms. (See the Enzymes chapter.)

Here's how prometabolic eating helps you control your blood sugar and insulin levels. When you fast, or undereat, or eat small amounts of natural foods (low-carb), your pancreas secretes the hormone glucagon, and your insulin level drops. When glucagon dominates the scene, your body's energy is derived from its stored sugar (glycogen) and fat reserve—so by encouraging glucagon dominance, you're turning your body into a fat-burning machine. Fat burns slowly and provides long-lasting energy, and you lose weight.

Also, when insulin drops, your level of growth hormone (GH) can rise. That is desirable, because GH rejuvenates and repairs tissues, which is anti-aging. During the day, GH secretion is usually inhibited by a high-carb diet and the resulting high insulin secretion and fatigue.

In a nutshell, I'm encouraging you to eat like a hunter-gatherer. Undereat by having only small amounts of food during the day so as not to cause fatigue or any digestive difficulties during your active working hours, and then eat your largest meal when you're hungry in the early evening. During the day, eat living foods: fruits, soaked seeds and nuts, raw veggies, and berries. This low-carb diet supports both anabolism and catabolism. If you're super-hungry, at first have some yogurt, freshly made vegetable juices, and some more protein; avocadoes and soaked nuts are also good for excessive hunger. For your evening meal, eat raw veggies first, then proteins, then carbs. The fiber will fill you, insulin will be secreted in moderation rather than in a drastic spike, and you will not overburden your body with wastes and toxins.

All foods are not created equal. Some of the best vegetables are broccoli, cauliflower, cabbage, kale, and Brussels sprouts. If you eat fish, meats, eggs, and cheese, make sure they're organic. Seaweeds, bok choy, and dandelion leaf are high-energy foods. The safest carbs are root vegetables (but not potatoes), beans in moderation, carrots, pumpkin, and squashes. Don't overdo bananas, dates, and figs, as they spike insulin. Sauerkraut is excellent for supporting intestinal functions. If you live in a cold climate or if you tend to get cold, the thermogenics of warm steamed foods will help; miso and vegetable soups and broths are good for this.

As you eat smaller amounts of food, your body will detoxify naturally. You may experience a runny nose, some fatigue, fever, maybe even a skin rash. These are all normal manifestations of detoxifying. The cleaner the body becomes, the more efficient it becomes, and the better it absorbs nutrients—resulting in improved nutrition and fewer food cravings.

After one or two months, you will naturally adjust to this way of eating. When you follow the guidelines above to control your hunger, eat right, and let your metabolic and hormonal cycles work properly, your life will change. During the day, with your insulin down, glucagon and GH up, and pancreatic enzymatic secretions reduced, you'll be energized, creative, and happy. At night, you will sleep like a baby. What a great life, all under your control! Self-monitoring and eating the prometabolic way are just about all you need to set your life in motion. I promise you you'll find yourself in a better place—"a good place to hang out," as my children would say.

The Athlete

An athletic person who trains hard needs more nutrients: specifically, more protein, carbs, vitamins, and minerals. Watch out for too much protein, though, as that can stress the liver and kidneys. Your pH will tell you if you're too acidic. This means you're not digesting your protein, you're eating too much protein, or you're using the wrong kinds.

Steroids are no way to go. They throw your natural cycles off. Does it make sense to overstimulate and overrule nature within? Whatever you do in excess will cause a deficiency somewhere else down the line. For instance, if you take testosterone, your adrenal glands will say, "Why should we produce testosterone? It's being shot into the body artificially, so we'll just stop producing it." The law of cause and effect is always working.

I've described how to observe and support your hormonal activity by using the monitoring system in this book. Remember, when you're monitoring your blood pressure, you're monitoring the activity of your adrenals, which secrete several hormones, including testosterone, progesterone, DHEA, and estrogen. If your blood pressure is low, you may be deficient in these hormones. Keep your adrenals strong, and you'll always be an athlete.

Foundational Nutrition and the Energy of Foods

It's up to us to take care of ourselves and, when we're not well, to find the right doctor who can investigate the problem and prescribe the proper treatments. But what can we do for ourselves? Can you know what is good for you without having a medical degree? The answer is yes. Eating the proper foods is your first line of defense. And one thing is certain: you need fruits and vegetables. It has been proven that fruits and vegetables contain all the vitamins and minerals that the body needs, as well as numerous phytochemicals with many nutritional and protective properties.

I am not saying you can live on these foods alone, but they should definitely be included as a large part of everybody's diet. Among the most nutrient-dense vegetables are kale, parsley, cabbage, beets, and spinach, to name just a few. Berries and other fruits are vital foods for your body as well. Let me also remind you of the particular importance of raw foods. Most diseases are not genetic; rather, they are caused by toxicity or nutritional deficiencies—deficiencies in phytochemicals, enzymes, vitamins, minerals, or fatty acids, or in the nutrients we haven't discovered yet. This is one reason why we must eat a percentage of our food in the raw state, before it has lost its nutritional value to processing and cooking.

In addition, you can support any weakened body functions with specific herbs and whole-food supplements. Many people also benefit from taking digestive enzymes with meals and taking probiotics to support digestion and bowel activities. Specific vitamin, mineral, and other supplements can also be added to sustain the body's general health or to address a specific condition being treated.

The health food industry has recently realized that concentrated food sources are sometimes more bioavailable, or more easily absorbed by the body, than individual vitamins and minerals. Some supplement companies, to improve the absorption of their vitamin and mineral products, are now combining these nutrients with concentrated food powders. This is not to downplay the necessity of supplementation; rather, it is another important aspect of nutritional enhancement. Among these aspects, number one is finding the right supplement for the individual, and number two is making sure the supplement can be utilized by that individual's body.

There are two levels of value in foods. One level is the physical nutrients contained in the foods; the other is the energy level of the food by itself. A term that has been coined is "the energetics of foods"—that is, the electrons and molecular make-up of foods. Everything is energy. Remember high school chemistry class, when we were told that everything is made up of electrons, which make up molecules, which combine to make up the physical universe? It's the same with foods. And the more food is processed and cooked, the more the energetics of the food are destroyed.

Years ago, I was inspired by the power in natural, whole foods to develop Juice Plus+®, which is now sold and distributed by NSA, Inc. and has become the best-selling line of encapsulated fruit and vegetable products in the world. Juice Plus+® works well in several ways: it has been proven to be bioavailable, to improve digestion, and to increase the levels of phytochemicals, vitamins, and minerals in the bloodstream. One of the major reasons for these benefits is that Juice Plus+® powders are nutrient-dense, predigested supplements with enzymes added. Another reason is that the ratio of combined fruits and vegetables makes them easy to absorb. Furthermore, Juice Plus+® powders contain the phytochemicals from every food source that's in their formulas.

In his best-selling book *Nutripoints*, Dr. Roy Vartabedian presents the overall nutritional value of thousands of foods based on an analysis of 26 key nutrients. This analysis determines each food's Nutripoint score in a range of 0–100, reflecting the food's nutrient density, or nutrition per calorie; the higher the score, the better. (For details on Nutripoints calculations, see www.Nutripoints.com.) In his evaluation of the ingredients in Juice Plus+® capsules, he found that the formula's fruits, vegetables, and grains yielded up to five times the nutrient density of the average, fruit, vegetable or grain. Dr. Vartabedian states that Juice Plus+®

is just about the most nutrient-dense of any naturally occurring foods he has analyzed. *(Vartabedian R, Matthews K. Nutripoints. Designs for Wellness Press, Carlsbad, CA, 2007.)*

The various knock-off products on the market don't have the supporting research base that NSA has established. (See the Juice Plus+® chapter.) Primary research has been done for Juice Plus+®, as opposed to "borrowed research" in which information is given on the effects of each separate plant or other constituent in a product's formula, but no research has been conducted on the whole formula combined. Knowing about each separate fruit or vegetable or herb in a formula doesn't mean the combination is going to work as stated—research should be done on the whole formula as embodied in the product.

When you buy any supplement or other health product, look for primary research or similar information that proves its efficacy. Get your money's worth. Simply throwing a bunch of foods or nutrients into a capsule and calling it a nutritional supplement, without considering the energy aspect of each ingredient and their ratio to each other, is called "poly-pharmacy." It looks good on paper, but does it work when it's taken into the body? Don't be fooled by poly-pharmacy or borrowed research. Go with what has been proven.

Some natural remedies, of course, have proven their effectiveness over hundreds of years—maybe not scientifically, but by intuition and actual usage. Nowadays, however, we have technology at our disposal to prove the effectiveness of historically used plants, herbs, and homeopathic combinations. I've done energetics research on Juice Plus+® myself, using sensitive energy-measuring equipment. My formulas were used in clinical practice for ten years before NSA brought them to the marketplace on a large scale. The ancient Greek physician Hippocrates was correct when he said, "Let food be your medicine and medicine be your food."

Natural Food Combining for Better pH

One dietary change we should all make is to eliminate junk food, because most of it is acid-forming. We would all benefit from eating fewer refined carbohydrates and eating more low-starch vegetables, too. At times when you really want carbs, try eating high-starch vegetables. Sprouted grains are usually all right, but even these should be kept at a minimum. There are obviously foods that we shouldn't eat regularly; however, I'm sure that if you're balanced, indulging in them once in a while won't hurt you. You make your own choices. Let your pH be your guide.

If you're healthy, you won't have to follow the food combining instructions below to a T. But if you're trying to balance your pH, they will help.

Basic Food Combining Rules

1. Combine leafy green vegetables, non-starchy vegetables, and sprouts with only one other allowed category at one meal.

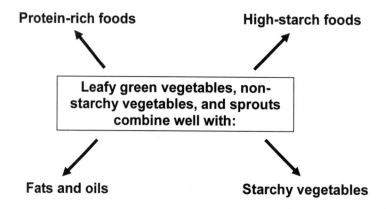

2. Avoid combining fruits and vegetables at one meal.

3. Avoid combining acid fruits with sweet fruits at one meal.

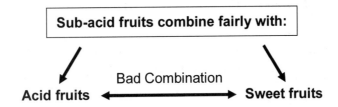

4. Eat melons alone.

The following lists will help you in proper food combining by identifying the foods that fall within each category.

PROTEIN-RICH FOODS
Combine Best with Leafy Green and Non-Starchy Vegetables

• DAIRY

• EGGS

• FISH

• MEAT

• NUTS: except for acorns and chestnuts, it is best to eat nuts raw after soaking them in water for eight hours or overnight.
Note: some nuts are also in the Fats category.
Note: peanuts are not actually nuts but legumes, and although they are a protein source, they are very difficult to digest; they are also in the High-Starch category.

Acorns (dried)	Filberts
Almonds	Hazelnuts
Beechnuts	Hickory nuts
Brazil nuts	Macadamia nuts
Butternuts	Pecans
Candlenuts	Pine nuts
Cashews	Pistachios
Chestnuts (dried)	Walnuts

• POULTRY

- SEEDS: eat raw or sprouted.
    Flaxseeds
    Pumpkin seeds
    Sesame seeds
    Sunflower seeds
- MISCELLANEOUS
    Brewer's yeast
    Nutritional yeast
    Dried beans
    Dried peas
    Miso
    Olives

FATS AND OILS
Combine Best with Leafy Green and Non-Starchy Vegetables

- AVOCADOS
- FATS:
    Butter
    Cheese
    Cream (heavy or light)
    Fatty meats
    Lard
    Margarine (avoid)
    Tallow
    Vegetable shortening (avoid)
- HYDROGENATED OILS: AVOID THESE.
- MOST NUTS: it is best to eat nuts raw after soaking them in water for eight hours or overnight.
    Brazil nuts
    Butternuts
    Candlenuts
    English walnuts
    Filberts
    Hickory nuts
    Pecans
    Pine nuts

• OILS: use cold-pressed oils only.
    Coconut oil (for cooking)
    Flax oil (never heat)
    Nut oils
    Olive oil
    Sesame oil
    Sunflower oil

HIGH-STARCH FOODS AND SUGARS
Combine Best with Leafy Green and Non-starchy Vegetables

• BREADS: sprouted or Essene breads are best.
• CEREALS AND GRAINS: eat cooked or sprouted. It is best to soak grains overnight in water mixed with an acidic liquid such as whey, lemon juice, or apple cider vinegar, before cooking them (exceptions are brown and wild rice).
    Amaranth
    Barley
    Buckwheat
    Kamut
    Millet
    Oats
    Quinoa
    Rice (brown or wild)
    Rye
    Sorghum
    Spelt
• DRIED BEANS AND PEAS: eat cooked or sprouted.
    Adzuki beans
    Chick peas/garbanzos
    Kidney beans
    Lima beans
    Peas (green or split)
    Pinto beans
• PASTAS: best to avoid.
    Spinach
    Spirulina
    Vegetable
• PEANUTS: very difficult to digest.

• POPCORN
• SYRUPS AND SUGARS: best to avoid.
    Brown sugar
    Candy
    Cane sugar or syrup
    Carob (roasted or raw)
    Chocolate
    Date sugar
    Fructose
    Honey (raw)
    Maple sugar
    Milk sugar
    Molasses (blackstrap)

STARCHY VEGETABLES
Combine best with Leafy Green and Non-Starchy Vegetables

• Eat cooked or raw:
    Artichoke
    Beet
    Carrot
    Cauliflower
    Corn – not recommended
    Jerusalem artichoke
    Mushroom
    Parsnip
    Potato – not recommended
    Pumpkin
    Rutabaga
    Salsify (a wild root vegetable)
    Sweet potato
    Winter squash (acorn, butternut, banana, Hubbard, and the like)
    Yam

LEAFY GREEN AND NON-STARCHY VEGETABLES
Combine best with Proteins, Fats and Oils, Starches, and Starchy Vegetables
• Eat cooked or raw:

Asparagus
Bamboo shoots
Beet greens
Broccoli
Brussels sprouts
Buckwheat lettuce
Cabbage (white, red,
  or Chinese)
Celery
Chicory
Chives
Collard greens
Cowslips
Cucumber
Dandelion greens
Eggplant
Endive
Escarole
Garlic
Green beans
Kale
Kohlrabi
Leafy greens
Leek

Lettuce (Bibb, Boston,
  Green/red-leaf, romaine)
Mint
Mullein
Mustard greens
Okra
Onion
Parsley
Peppers (red or green)
Radish
Radish greens
Rhubarb
Scallion
Seaweed (dulse, kelp, nori,
  wakame, and the like)
Sorrel
Spinach
Summer squash
Sunflower greens
Swiss chard
Turnip greens
Watercress
Weeds
Wheatgrass
Zucchini

• SPROUTS: eat raw, do not cook.
Alfalfa sprouts
Broccoli sprouts
Cabbage sprouts
Fenugreek sprouts
Lentil sprouts
Mung bean sprouts
Mustard seed sprouts
Radish sprouts
Red clover sprouts

SUB-ACID FRUITS
Combine fairly with Acid and Sweet Fruits

Apple
Apricot
Blueberries
Cherimoya
Fresh figs
Grapes
Guava
Huckleberries
Kiwi fruit

Mango
Nectarine
Papaya
Pear
Sweet apple
Sweet cherries
Sweet peach
Sweet plum

ACID FRUITS
Combine fairly with Sub-Acid Fruits

Blackberries
Grapefruit
Kumquat
Lemon
Lime
Orange
Pineapple
Pomegranate
Raspberries

Sour apple
Sour cherries
Sour grapes
Sour peach
Sour plum
Strawberries
Tangerine
Tomato
Ugli fruit

SWEET FRUITS
Combine fairly with Sub-Acid Fruits

Banana (dried or fresh)
Currants
Dates (dried or fresh)
Dried fruit – always
   soak before eating
Figs
Muscat grapes
Peach

Persimmon
Plum
Prune
Raisins
Sweet apple
Sweet cherries
Thompson grapes

MELONS
Combine badly with all other foods—best to eat alone

Banana melon
Cantaloupe
Casaba melon
Christmas melon
Crenshaw melon
Honey-ball melon
Honeydew melon
Watermelon

Rules to Aid Digestion

Helping your body digest its foods properly is one of the best things you can do for your health. In Part Two of this book, you learned how using the monitoring system to improve your digestion can help balance your terrain. Here are some additional tips:

• Avoid drinking liquids twenty minutes before meals, during meals, and for one hour following meals, as liquids dilute the digestive juices and hinder digestion.

• Avoid drinking liquids that are too cold (out of the refrigerator or with ice) or too hot (close to boiling), because these temperature extremes stress the digestive system and may cause indigestion.

• Because most dessert items do not combine well with foods eaten at meals, it is best to avoid them.

• Avoid eating immediately before or after strenuous exercise.

• If possible, avoid eating during acute episodes of extreme physical or mental distress.

• Thoroughly chew and salivate all foods.

• Avoid overeating.

• Avoid eating three to four hours before bedtime. Especially avoid eating fruit at night, because it's very stimulating and can disturb sleep.

CHOOSING THE RIGHT DIET AND SUPPLEMENTS FOR YOU

The foundation for achieving and maintaining your optimal health is to discover, and then follow, the best diet for your unique body and its needs. Metabolic, vegan, high-protein, low-carbohydrate, whatever—the monitoring system will tell you what's working for you and what isn't.

As you begin this exploration, consider the dietary mistakes in the 1970s and 80s. A vegetarian diet, for instance, was shown to be healing and cleansing for people with cancer. A cancer patient's internal terrain is way out of balance and usually very acidic. Vegetarianism is great for such a person—as a short-term therapeutic measure. The mistake was thinking that vegetarianism was good for everybody all the time. I found out differently, from personal experience and in my practice; I have seen too many anemic, amino-acid-deficient vegetarians. Many have since gone back to eating lean, organic meats, and now they look and feel wonderful.

When the Pritikin diet came along, the very high-carbohydrate and very low-fat regime sounded promising at first. Over a period of time, however, its flaws became apparent. That way of eating can lead to Syndrome X, over-secretion of insulin, and pancreatic problems. (See the Insulin chapter.)

Next came the macrobiotic diet, also a high-carb regime, which entails eating mostly cooked food and very little raw food. Again, this diet was promoted because of its initial positive results for people with cancer. But remember, cancer patients are very sick, and even a little bit of good nutrition can go a long way for a weakened system full of toxins.

My first point in these examples is that all diets—not just the unhealthful fad diets—have had their failures. One size does not fit all. And my second point is that when you're choosing a diet, you want that diet to have been studied in healthy people, not just sick people. Fortunately, such research does exist.

In the 1930s, the visionary dentist Weston A. Price traveled the world to study the dentition of healthy people in isolated cultures untouched by Western civilization and its foods. He found that these peoples invariably had great bone structure, wide dental arches, and beautiful straight teeth—along with exceptional health, due in large measure to native diets rich in nutrient-dense foods, fat-soluble vitamins, and animal proteins.

Dr. Price also documented what happened to the dental and physical health of these peoples as introduced Western foods displaced the native diets: these dietary changes led to a dramatic decline in health within one generation. *(Price WA. Nutrition and Physical Degeneration, 6th ed. Keats Publishing, New Canaan, CT, 2003.)* (A Web site sponsored by a foundation carrying on Price's work and legacy, www.westonaprice.org, provides a wealth of great articles, a quarterly magazine on nutrition and health, and information on buying organic foods throughout the country.)

Many books claim that a given diet helped some people who were ill. But most of the time, sick people and healthy people have different dietary needs—so I want to look at both sides of that coin. Will a diet that works well for a sick person also meet the nutritional requirements of a healthy individual, a growing child, an athlete, or an elderly person? This issue is one of the reasons that I felt it was important to develop a monitoring system to help people make intelligent choices about their personal nutrition.

Following the latest diet trend or imitating an exotic nutrition practice may, or may not, be right for you. Whatever the diet is that catches your interest, investigate by looking at research conducted on the diet. Then, if you decide to try it, you can monitor its effects to assess whether it's suitable for you. You can't know what the future will bring, but you do know what your pH, temperature, and blood pressure should be. These health indicators speak to you in a language you can interpret and respond to accordingly.

Foods today are often nutrient-deficient, and any given individual may have a longstanding deficiency, or be under an unusual amount of stress, or work out a lot, or have an acute or chronic illness. Even a diet that is generally good for you might not provide enough of one or more specific nutrients to bring you into your own optimal balance. For example, you might have found the right diet but are still deficient in iodine, manifesting as a low body temperature reflecting reduced thyroid function. The monitoring system tells you "where you're at" and helps you make the necessary corrections to bring you back into balance. Dietary supplements can be very helpful in this regard—and can also have many beneficial effects against illnesses and disorders.

This chapter is intended to introduce you (or reintroduce you) to various important food groups and nutrient factors. There's a lot to consider in making informed food choices and designing the diet that is right for you, but the results—your best health and well-being—are well worth it.

Basic Foods and Other Fundamentals

I never like to be rigid with dietary "rules" because chances are that people won't stick to them. If you're healthy and strong, and you indulge once in a while and then get back on track, my attitude is, "So what?" For instance, during the Christmas holiday season, if one of my clients brings me a gift of "cookies baked with love," then move over, Rover—I'm going to have a few, and love it, and I'm not going to condemn myself. We all know that self-criticism is more destructive than a cookie.

Start with what we know for certain: we all need water and fresh vegetables and fruits; lean meats are a good protein source; seeds, nuts, and sprouted grains are additional good options; and unhealthy fats, sugars, excessive alcohol, overprocessed baked goods, and fried foods should be avoided as much as possible or eliminated entirely. Now how hard can it be to subtract the negatives and monitor your body's response to the positives that remain? Have fun with it. It's an intelligent way to travel.

After a while of healthful eating, you'll find your body craves the good foods it needs. I'm not suggesting any one-size-fits-all diet—and I'm not saying that you should or should not eat meat, or eggs, or what have you. These choices are all yours. What I am saying is that you should know about your foods and eat according to a diet that you feel is best for you.

Some general principles to keep in mind: Cooked and denatured foods, especially flesh foods and acid-forming simple sugars, spike insulin secretion. Flesh foods can putrefy in the intestines, and sugars can ferment. These imbalances disturb the body's pH and lower its vitality. Acidifying foods rob your body of its much-needed alkaline minerals. Acidification also allows your terrain to support the growth of molds and yeast that secrete harmful mycotoxins.

(You probably already have a half-dozen recipe books, but I'd like to recommend one of my favorites: *Nourishing Traditions* by Sally Fallon and Mary Enig, from New Trends Publishing, Inc. It's chock-full of information that will clarify many questions on foods.)

Vegetables. You should eat as many vegetables as possible—organic is best. All leafy green vegetables should be eaten raw. Root vegetables and other hard vegetables can be lightly steamed or juiced; the cooking frees fiber-bound nutrients and helps warm the body in a cold climate.

The family of cruciferous vegetables, including broccoli, kale, Brussels sprouts, and cauliflower, contain important anticancer phytochemicals such as indole-3 carbinol. They also help the liver detoxify potentially problematic substances such as estrogen derivatives and chemicals called xenoestrogens. (See the Phytochemicals chapter.)

Eat as much green food as possible. Chlorophyll helps purify your blood, build red blood cells, and increase oxygen levels in your body.

(Chlorophyll is further discussed below.) "If you're not green inside, you're not clean inside!"

Fruits. Fruits are good foods that contain vitamins and minerals plus fiber. Fruit is best eaten as the whole food rather than as fruit juice, because fruit juice is so highly concentrated with sugars. (Juice Plus+® is an exception, as the sugar is removed.) Fruit is better eaten in a warm climate, as it is a cooling food; also, in this situation it is more likely to have ripened naturally and traveled less distance to your store.

If fruit sugars cause a problem in your system, your pH will reflect an acidic reaction. Take your salivary and urinary pH before a fruit meal, then repeat your readings two hours afterward, and you'll know whether fruit sugars are an issue.

Usually keeping fruit at about 5 percent of your diet is all right, unless you have a sugar-metabolism problem such as diabetes. If you have a thyroid or adrenal problem, monitor your fruit intake carefully. (See the chart in the Thyroid and Adrenal chapter.) Avoid fruit altogether if you have Candida.

Meat, poultry, and eggs. If you choose to eat meat and/or poultry, make sure it's organic and grass-fed if possible. Grain-fed animals are usually higher in fat and their feed is laced with herbicides and pesticides. Organic poultry, lamb, beef, ostrich, turkey, and buffalo are good choices. Eat small amounts and always take digestive enzymes before your meal.

Animals experience tremendous fear and stress due to inhumane treatment and the way they're slaughtered. This causes large secretions of adrenaline, which is then metabolized into a compound called adrenochrome, which can destroy muscle tissue in your body. This, plus the antibiotics and hormones animals are injected with, accumulate in your intestinal tract and cause bacterial imbalance just as if you were taking the antibiotics yourself. This is another reason why, if you eat flesh foods, it's so important to eat fresh vegetables and take probiotics daily. (Probiotics are described below.)

Organic eggs are best. And you can eat the whole egg, not just the white—cholesterol isn't the villain it's been portrayed to be.

Fish. If possible, fish should be wild-caught and fresh. Low-fat white fish such as sole and flounder is a good choice. The essential fatty acids (EFAs) in fish are important for brain function and for every cell in your body. These EFAs are also precursors for prostaglandins and other hormones. Unfortunately, a lot of fish is contaminated with mercury and other toxins from polluted waters. (If you're using fish oil, call the manufacturer and ask for a print-out of the heavy metal content in the product.)

Essential fats. A very low-fat diet can have a detrimental effect on the health and functioning of both body and brain. You need some fat in your diet to serve as building blocks for hormones and other substances, to serve crucial functions in cell membranes, and to ensure the body's absorption of fat-soluble nutrients. Specific fatty acids can also be very helpful against inflammatory conditions and other disease states. It is important to be able to distinguish between the types of fats so you can eat the right ones and avoid the harmful ones. (See the Fats chapter.)

Researchers have found that omega-3 fatty acids (from fish, fish oils, walnut oil, and flaxseed oil) help prevent inflammatory conditions such as lupus, asthma, and arthritic conditions. Omega-3s have also been used for Crohn's disease, ulcerative colitis, and irritable bowel syndrome. Whenever there is an inflammatory condition in your body, increase your omega-3 intake and increase omega-6s (from seed oils, corn oil, olive oil, sunflower oil, and safflower oil) to keep them in the ideal 1:1 ratio.

The brain's major constituent, other than water, is fat—60 percent. With sufficient amounts of omega-3s in the diet, the membranes surrounding your brain cells can perform their crucial roles in your cognitive abilities and mental health. But without sufficient omega-3s, brain cell membranes must substitute omega-6 and monounsaturated fatty acids, which have totally different properties. Researchers have linked omega-3 deficiency to depression, anxiety, and bipolar disorder.

Dietary fiber. Fiber is actually several substances contained in plant cell walls: cellulose (in wheat bran), hemicellulose (in oat bran), gums (such as gum arabic), mucilages (guar), pectins (in citrus rind and apple), algin and carageenan (in seaweed), and lignans (in flaxseed, cabbage, wheat, and apple). Vegetables, fruits, and whole grains are excellent fiber sources.

Dietary fiber speeds the transit time of bowel movements by bulking up the stool; it is sometimes used for constipation, and this same effect also helps against intestinal acidification. The longer your waste products stay in your colon, the more opportunity exists for fermentation and acidification; these acids are then absorbed into the blood. Intestinal acidification can be a major stumbling block when you're working to balance your terrain.

Having enough fiber in the diet is therefore of bottom-line importance no matter what your state of health may be. Diseases and conditions associated with a low-fiber diet are constipation, appendicitis, diverticulosis, hemorrhoids, colon cancer, irritable bowel syndrome, ulcerative colitis, and Crohn's disease.

Cellulose does not dissolve in water; rather, it absorbs water and thereby increases the size and weight of the stool. It is partially digested by bacteria in the intestines and releases several useful short-chain fatty acids. Propionic acid and acetic acid, for example, go to the liver and are used for energy. Butyric acid becomes butyrate, an important energy source for the cells in the colon wall.

The non-cellulose, mucilaginous fibers such as oat bran, guar gum, and pectins are water-soluble. They bind with excess fats and cholesterol in the intestines, escorting them out of the body through the stool and lowering serum cholesterol. The water-insoluble fibers have less effect on serum cholesterol, and wheat bran may produce intestinal irritation in some people. Various fiber products are available at health food stores.

Beans. Pinto beans, kidney beans, black beans, adzuki, white beans, lentils, and all peas are examples of this food group. Dried beans are typically fresher in a health food store than in a regular grocery store. Avoid canned beans, because their enzymes have been destroyed by the heat involved in canning.

Eat beans only in moderation. Their starch is one of the main reasons you want to limit their use. They are best eaten sprouted: soak for eight hours, then rinse and cook them slowly. There is some controversy about soybeans and soy products; they should not be used in excess, as they contain estrogen-like substances that can be troublesome. (See www.SoyOnlineService.co.nz.)

Grains. The grain products in your diet should be 100 percent whole grain and preferably sprouted first. You can buy sprouted-grain bread at your health food store. The sprouting process (soaking grains overnight and then letting them sit for four to eight hours) begins to predigest them. Their own enzymes start to break down the protein, fats, and carbohydrates into simpler forms, releasing some of the enzyme inhibitors grains contain and making them easier to digest. But keep grain consumption at a minimum, and check your pH after eating them to see their effect on your terrain.

Processed grain-based foods should be avoided, as they are typically made of refined white flour from which the grain's nutritious bran and germ have been removed. Many inflammatory diseases and pancreatic problems have manifested with the advent of diets based increasingly on refined grains. Grains have a high concentration of carbohydrates, which can overburden your digestive system's absorption ability. A diet high in refined carbohydrates causes many problems: for example, a disease cluster called Syndrome X that includes type II diabetes, hyperinsulinism, insulin resistance, and hypoglycemia. (See the Insulin chapter.) Avoid grains if you have any pancreatic problems.

Grain products include cereals, popcorn, crackers, rice cakes, cookies, cakes, muffins, bagels, pancakes, and many more. It's helpful to use digestive enzymes (described below) when eating these concentrated starches. Never eat grains that have been stored for long periods, as they begin to ferment and develop fungus.

(A book you may find interesting is Dr. Joseph Mercola's *The No-Grain Diet*, published by Dutton. Please note that when I mention a book, that doesn't necessarily mean I agree with everything in it; and of course, the ultimate choice of what to agree with and what to do is always yours.)

Milk products. Unless they are organic, milk and milk products contain pesticides, herbicides, hormones, and antibiotics. Also, during pasteurization, their enzymes are denatured or altered by the heat, which means they are essentially deactivated—and that's not all. Up to 90 percent of milk's unsaturated fatty acids are also destroyed. Dr. Karen Jenson reports that pasteurization transforms the cow's milk protein called casein into a chemical called percaseinate, which combines with calcium and prevents its absorption. Lysine, an amino acid important for strong teeth and bones, is destroyed as well. Surprise!

Try almond or rice milk instead of pasteurized cow's milk. Organic, unprocessed goat's milk is another option. You should, however, limit your use of soy milk. (See www.SoyOnlineService.co.nz.) If you do use cow's milk products, keep them at a minimum. People who are lactose intolerant should avoid milk products altogether.

Simple carbohydrates (sugar and starch). All sugars and starches can turn into fat in the body. Refined sugars including dextrose, fructose, galactose, honey, sugar cane, and sorghum raise blood glucose levels rapidly and throw your body into a very stressful insulin situation. (See the Insulin chapter.) Starches are highly concentrated carbohydrates that are difficult to digest; they are broken down into simple sugars, so the same insulin effect results from eating sugars or starches. Furthermore, sugar ferments in the intestinal tract and can trigger fungal growth.

Complex carbohydrates in whole foods with fiber take longer to digest and are more effective at maintaining your energy. Keep in mind, though, that your body is still using insulin to utilize or store these sugars.

If you have or suspect any glandular imbalance, check your temperature and blood pressure after eating any sugary food. If you have Candida or any digestive problem, avoid sugar. Obviously, people who have diabetes or other sugar-metabolism problems such as hypoglycemia should avoid sugar as well. So please limit your sugar—but you can have a Christmas cookie.

Yeast. If possible, avoid yeast, baked goods that contain yeast, and other yeasted products, or use them sparingly. These include brewer's yeast, baker's yeast, and nutritional yeast. I don't see any sense in eating these microforms, as their secreted mycotoxins can cause acidifying reactions and yeast overgrowth in your body.

Corn, corn products, and peanuts. If possible, avoid these or use them sparingly. These products can contain fungus and fungal byproducts. They are also difficult to digest.

Microwaving. Most microwaved foods have an acidifying effect on the body. Russian research has shown that microwaving food destroys enzymes, renders vitamins and minerals unabsorbable, and creates harmful free radicals. It is suspected that microwaving foods can increase certain cancers. Avoid microwaved foods entirely.

Artificial sweeteners. Avoid the aspartames of the world. They are acid-forming and considered to be neurotoxins (poisons that irritate the nerve sheaths). Artificial sweeteners have been linked to symptoms such as dizziness, vertigo, depression, fatigue, heart irregularities, ringing in the ears, anxiety, joint pain—the list goes on. Substances like this can aggravate any illness.

Probiotics. These "friendly" bacteria are normally present in your intestinal tract and are a vital aid to digestion. Probiotic supplements are usually used to combat Candida or other fungal problems. The most widely used and most well-researched probiotics are *Lactobacillus acidophilus* and *Bifidobacterium bifidum.* Antibiotics destroy harmful and friendly bacteria at the same time, so if you have taken antibiotics, take probiotics to replace your natural bacterial population. I recommend using the dairy versions of probiotic supplements.

Enzymes. Digestive enzymes help you get the most nutrition out of the foods you eat. Raw foods contain many of the enzymes that help digest them. I recommend supplemental enzymes to everyone who eats cooked food. Digestive enzyme supplements are also used to eliminate gas, bloating, fermentation, and intestinal upset. (See the Enzymes chapter.)

Chlorophyll. All life energy comes from the sun. Green plants possess the ability to capture solar energy and store it in chlorophyll molecules, to be passed on up the food chain. This "blood" of plants is a lot like our blood, because chlorophyll bears a striking resemblance to the oxygen-bearing red pigment hemoglobin. A hemoglobin molecule is a web of carbon, hydrogen, oxygen, and nitrogen atoms grouped around an atom of iron; chlorophyll is a similar web but with a centerpiece of magnesium.

The famed Swiss physician Dr. Max Bircher-Benner claimed chlorophyll strengthens the heart, arteries, intestines, uterus, and lungs.

Dr. Benjamine Gurskin treated more than 1,000 patients suffering from intestinal inflammations, head colds, and sinus infections with chlorophyll, and recorded that every single case was either improved or cured. *(Gurskin B. Am J Surg 1940 49:49.)* Green juices are excellent for most intestinal problems and inflammations. Liquid chlorophyll can be taken between meals for throat and intestinal inflammations, colitis, and enteritis.

You can purchase liquid chlorophyll at health food stores or make your own green juice at home. If you have a juicer, try a green drink of romaine lettuce, parsley, celery, perhaps kale, and a little apple. Many of these vital whole foods are ingredients in Juice Plus+®. (See the Juice Plus+® chapter.)

Anti-Inflammatory Supplements and Herbs

This section describes non-foundational supplements and herbs that should be taken only as specifically needed. It's advisable to be professionally monitored when using non-foundational supplements and to take them for no more than two weeks at a time, unless recommended otherwise by your healthcare professional.

Proteolytic enzymes. Proteolytic enzymes (also called proteases) break down proteins into amino acids. Some of the best known are pancreatic proteases, chymotrypsin and trypsin, bromelain (from pineapple), papain (from papaya), and fungal proteases. (See the Enzymes chapter.)

Proteolytic enzymes help the immune system by breaking down antigen-antibody complexes that form during infections and autoimmune diseases. They have a long history of use in cancer treatment as well as for inflammations, swellings, and pain. Proteolytic enzymes have been used to treat conditions including myofascial pain syndrome, fibromyalgia, sport injuries, lupus, arthritis, circulatory problems, and all infections. Use them immediately for colds, fever, and respiratory or sinus mucous conditions. Take them after a tooth extraction to reduce pain and swelling.

When proteolytic enzymes are used therapeutically, they are taken in large doses between meals so as not to interfere with, or be delayed by, digestion. You want them to be absorbed quickly from the gastrointestinal tract and carried through the bloodstream to the treatment site. An excessively acidic or alkaline terrain can affect enzymes' reaction rates or even render them inactive, so it's important to monitor your pH for optimum effectiveness when using them. (Let me refer you to several good books: _Food Enzymes: The Missing Link to Radiant Health_, by Humbart Santillo, from Hohm Press; _The Complete Book of Enzyme Therapy_, by Anthony Cichoke, from Avery Publishing Group; _The Enzyme Cure_, by Lita Lee and Lisa Turner, from Future Medicine Publishing; and _Enzyme Nutrition_, by Edward Howell, from Avery Publishing Group.)

Methylsulfonylmethane (MSM). MSM is a water-soluble, non-metallic sulfur compound. Sulfur is one of the most common elements in the body, with its highest concentrations found in joints, hair, skin, nails, organs, and blood. It is also a component of insulin.

Sulfur is necessary for the formation of connective tissue, so supplemental MSM is used for all joint inflammatory problems to reduce joint degeneration and inflammation. Researchers claim that MSM can help with osteoarthritis, stiffness and swelling, circulation, pain, scar tissue, calcium deposits, rheumatoid arthritis, lupus, sinus infection, allergy, asthma, gum disease, and hyperacidity of the stomach and intestines. _(Jacob S, Lawrence R. The Miracle of MSM: The Natural Solution for Pain. G.P. Putnam's Sons, New York, NY, 1999.)_ It also reduces lactic acid buildup, which is a helpful effect for athletes and exercisers.

The daily dosage range for MSM is 2–20 grams. It's important to be professionally monitored while you are taking MSM. Most professionals agree that MSM should only be used in a short-term therapeutic approach of less than two weeks' duration. MSM is often taken in combination with glucosamine sulfate (described below).

Glucosamine sulfate. Glucosaminoglycans (GAGs) are a category of substances that make up cartilage, connective tissue (including tendons, ligaments, and blood vessels), and bone. Glucosamine sulfate, the most researched of the GAG group, is best known for stimulating the synthesis of other GAGs within the joints. One of the reasons glucosamine sulfate is so effective is that its molecular size is much smaller than other GAGs, which helps it penetrate the joint capsule.

As we age, it appears that we lose the ability to manufacture sufficient glucosamine, which results in cartilage breakdown, degeneration of joint structure, and inflammatory joint disease like arthritis. Research has shown that long-term use of glucosamine sulfate produces better results than non-steroidal anti-inflammatory drugs (NSAIDs) at relieving pain and inflammation in joints and connective tissue; furthermore, it helps repair damaged joints.

Glucosamine sulfate is often found in combination with other GAGs. The usual dose of supplemental glucosamine sulfate is 500 milligrams taken three times daily. Make sure it is combined with MSM (described above), or take the two together. Any time you're dealing with joint problems, minerals such as zinc, copper, manganese, and boron are necessary in your diet as well. *(Murray ML, Pizzorno J. Encyclopedia of Natural Medicine. Prima Publishing, Rocklin, CA, 1998.)* Dr. Charles Cochran has developed an excellent product called Joint Health (866-798-7818). Another easily absorbed, elemental glucosamine sulfate supplement is Body High, from Reality Health (877-454-3313); along with predigested amino acids, it's a good addition when you're rebuilding tissue.

Bioflavonoids. In nature, vitamin C is found closely associated with bioflavonoids, which are synergistic substances that potentiate its action.

They strengthen blood vessel walls and reduce swelling, inflammation, and bleeding. Examples of widely used bioflavonoids are rutin (in buckwheat), hesperidin (in lemons and oranges), and quercetin (in quercetin bark, wild fruits, red clover blossoms, onions, and buckwheat). (See the Phytochemicals chapter.)

Bioflavonoids have been used for retinal hemorrhage prevention, bruising, bleeding of the gums, arthritis, herpes infection, arteriosclerosis, allergic response, inner ear problems, and inflammation after injury. If you take a vitamin C supplement for any inflammatory condition, make sure the formula includes bioflavonoids. Doses of bioflavonoids are 500–3,000 milligrams daily.

Turmeric. A common spice, turmeric has been used in Ayurvedic and Chinese medicine for centuries and is noted as a strong anti-inflammatory agent. Turmeric contains a yellow pigment called curcumin, which is anti-inflammatory itself and has been known to be as effective as cortisone in acute situations such as sprains, muscular pain, and inflamed joints. *(Arora R, et al. Anti-inflammatory studies on Curcuma longa (turmeric). Ind J Med Res 1971 59:1289-1295.)* Turmeric or curcumin is often used in combination with other anti-inflammatory agents.

Ginger. Ginger has a long history in the treatment of gastrointestinal ailments. It helps control digestive imbalances and inhibits blood platelet aggregation. Ginger also soothes the intestinal tract, relaxes the intestinal walls, and helps expel gas. Ginger acts as a carrier for other herbs and is usually found in combination formulas for inflammation or intestinal issues. Ginger root tea is excellent for an upset stomach: boil one ounce of the root for twenty minutes, steep for ten minutes, and drink throughout the day. Limit the time that you use ginger therapeutically to two weeks maximum.

Ginkgo. Ginkgo's primary therapeutic property is to increase blood flow into areas of the brain, the lower limbs, arteries, veins, and small capillaries. It has been used for conditions such as vertigo, tinnitus (ringing in the ears), hearing loss, circulatory problems, peripheral arterial insufficiency, dementia, and memory loss. Ginkgo's relevance to inflammation is that it supports the body's tissue repair process by promoting blood flow toward damaged or inflamed areas. It's often combined with other anti-inflammatory herbs to help them circulate to the area of disturbance. (*Murray ML. The Healing Power of Herbs. Prima Publishing, Rocklin, CA, 1995.*)

Boswellia. Historically, boswellia (also known as salai guggul) has been used to treat osteoarthritis. One of its basic "ingredients" is boswellic acid, a gum with anti-inflammatory properties. Boswellia extract is used as an anti-inflammatory agent for cartilage and joint problems. It has also been used for conditions such as colitis, ulcerative colitis, Crohn's disease, and asthma. (*PDR for Herbal Medicine, 1st ed. Medical Economics Company, Montvale, NJ, 1998.*)

Licorice. Licorice root (*Glycyrrhiza glabra*)—not the candy—is an excellent remedy for intestinal inflammation and ulcers. Licorice has been proven to be more effective than Tagamet and Zantac. (*Murray ML. The Healing Power of Herbs. Prima Publishing, Rocklin, CA, 1995.*) Research has shown 760 milligrams three times a day between meals to be an effective dose. *Caution:* Do not use licorice if you have high blood pressure. Avoid aspirin, NSAIDs, and corticosteroids when taking licorice.

Slippery elm bark, aloe vera, and marshmallow root. These herbs are very mucilaginous, which is why they soothe the intestinal tract and are so healing for gastrointestinal conditions. They're good for all bowel, stomach, and intestinal inflammations, irritable bowel syndrome, ulcers, and diarrhea. *(Christopher J. The School of Natural Healing. Bi-World Publishers, Provo, UT, 1976.)* They're also good for constipation. *Caution:* Do not use any herb in cases of intestinal blockage; if you've been diagnosed with such a blockage, follow your physician's advice.

These herbs are usually found in combination formulas. Taking them in tea form may speed their action against intestinal inflammation; several cups a day between meals are recommended.

White willow bark. White willow bark is often found in combination formulas with some of the above-mentioned herbs. It is used for musculoskeletal pain and arthritis. Certain salicylates are found in this herb, giving it analgesic and anti-inflammatory properties.

A note about nightshades. Dr. Norman Childers demonstrated that the Solonaceae family of plants, commonly called nightshades, crippled or even killed animals that grazed on them—and he cured his own arthritis by eliminating these plants from his diet. *(Childers NF, Russo GM. The Nightshades and Health. Horticultural Publications, New Brunswick, NJ, 1977.)* If you have any inflammatory condition, avoid the nightshades, which include tomatoes, potatoes, eggplant, peppers, and tobacco. They contain an alkaloid that inhibits normal collagen repair in the joints. One exception to this rule is cayenne pepper (section following), which seems to be helpful to some arthritics who are not allergic to the nightshades (if you have any questions about this, see your licensed health professional).

Cayenne pepper. The familiar hot red pepper cayenne (also called capsicum) is unequalled at normalizing blood circulation. It has been used for muscle pain, rheumatic conditions, arthritis, frostbite, gastrointestinal disorders, fevers, and arteriosclerosis. Cayenne is excellent for all mucous conditions and congestion, in which circulation must be increased for proper detoxification. It is good for increasing blood flow when taken alone or in combination formulas, in which it potentiates the effect of other herbs. You can use cayenne daily on foods or take ¼ teaspoon in water as a circulatory tonic. *(Murray ML. The Healing Power of Herbs. Prima Publishing, Rocklin, CA, 1995.)*

Herbs for the Liver

If your salivary pH is continually acidic, this indicates that your liver is retaining acids and needs support in order to do its job of detoxifying your body. Most herbs that restore liver function also support digestion; taken along with supplemental enzymes, they can be very helpful in correcting liver and intestinal dysfunctions and imbalances. Two excellent companies offering herbal combinations for the liver and gall bladder are Gaia Herbs (888-917-8269) and Herb Pharm (800-348-4372). Their products can be found in most health food stores.

Milk thistle. Known to protect the liver from damage and enhance detoxification, milk thistle is a strong antioxidant. For proper detoxification of harmful chemicals, the liver requires glutathione, and milk thistle prevents the depletion of glutathione in the liver. Milk thistle has been used to treat alcoholism, cirrhosis, chronic hepatitis, and fat buildup in the liver. (Drinking excessive amounts of alcohol depletes glutathione.) It is also excellent for gall bladder problems. Liquid extract of milk thistle is the best form to use.

Dandelion root and leaf. Dandelion has a strong positive effect on the liver, gall bladder, and digestive system, and it also has a positive effect on the kidneys. It has been used for recovery from hepatitis and liver and digestive disorders. This herb's additional effect on sugar metabolism has been utilized successfully in diabetes to keep blood sugar levels low. Dandelion is taken in tea, tincture, or capsule form.

Artichoke extract. Similarly to milk thistle, artichoke extract protects the liver from toxins' poisonous effects. It helps regenerate damaged liver cells, and over weeks of use it has significantly restored severely damaged livers. Artichoke extract reduces levels of cholesterol and other fats in the bloodstream by mobilizing fats for excretion from the body.

Research on artichoke extract has focused on its use in preventing atherosclerosis and serum cholesterol increase. It has also been used for gall bladder problems, jaundice, and digestive problems. *(Caruzzo C, et al. Considerazioni sull'attivita dell'acido 1,4-dicaffeilchinoco sulle frzioni lipidiche del siero nell'aterosclerosi. Minerva Med 1969 60:4514; Greten H, et al. Die lipoproteinelektrophorese zur diagnose von hyperlipoproteinaemian. Deutsche Medizinische Wochenschrift 1970 95:1716; Eberhardt G. Untersuchungen ueber die wirkung von cynabei leberzellvertettung. Z Gastroenterol 1973 11:183; Hammerl H, et al. Ueber den einfluss von cynarin auf hyperlipidaemien untr besonderer beruechsichtingung des typs II (hypercholesterinaemie). Wiener Medizinische Wochenschrift 1973 41:601.)*

Other Herbs and Nutritionals

Again, some of the following herbs and nutritionals are non-foundational supplements to be taken for no more than two weeks at a time unless recommended otherwise by your healthcare professional.

Ashwagandha. Ashwagandha (also called winter cherry or Indian ginseng) is used in the Ayurvedic system of medicine as an aphrodisiac, as a diuretic, and for treating memory loss. This herb is found in many tonics and formulas for promoting energy and sexual vitality. Both men and women can use it for rejuvenating bones, muscles, and other tissues, the adrenal glands, and the reproductive system.

Like Siberian ginseng (described below), ashwagandha is an adaptogenic herb, which means it helps the body maintain homeostasis and resist the negative effects of stress. It is especially good in conditions such as arthritis, hypertension, diabetes, immune dysfunction, and other debilitating diseases. *(Padmawar A. www.amrutaherbals.com)* Ashwagandha is also helpful for athletes who need strength and faster recovery from the physical stress of training.

Siberian ginseng. Siberian ginseng (*Eleutherococcus senticosus*, not the Asian species *Panax ginseng*) acts as a general tonic for the whole body, restoring energy and increasing mental and physical performance. It is called an adaptogenic herb because it normalizes bodily functions and enhances resistance to physical and chemical stress. It's also considered an anti-stress herb because it helps regulate adrenal function and reduces the body's alarm response, decreasing feelings of stress and anxiety. It offsets the effect of cortisol and enhances liver function.

When your monitoring shows a blood pressure issue, you can use Siberian ginseng to help balance your adrenals. For a person under stress—and who isn't?—or recovering from a lengthy illness, Siberian ginseng is an excellent choice. (See my book, *Natural Healing with Herbs*, from Hohm Press, for more information on herbs and detoxification.)

Mucuna. Mucuna has been reported to be a nerve tonic and a mild aphrodisiac and also has antioxidant qualities. This herb influences mood and sexuality and supports libido in aging individuals. Its active constituents include alkaloids, mucanine, pruridine, tannic acid, resin, lecithin, and most importantly, L-dopa, which the body uses to make the important neurotransmitter dopamine. *(www.ars-grin.gov.)* Mucuna has been used for generations in India to treat Parkinson's disease, for which it is being studied as a long-term treatment.

In addition to L-dopa, mucuna also contains the dopamine precursor levodopa. Dopamine production enhances testosterone activity, and anything that boosts dopamine in the brain could provide natural support and stimulation of sexual desire and enhancement. *(Giuliano F, Allard J. Dopamine and male sexual function. Eur Urol 2001 40:601-608; Giuliano F, Allard J. Dopamine and sexual function. Int J Impot Res 2001 suppl 3:S18-S28.)*

Mucuna is a perfect example of how herbs work in synchrony with the body. It's always a good idea to use whole foods and herbs to support body functions by supplying precursors for the body to make what it needs without overstimulation by drugs or synthetic hormones. This is what I call foundational nutrition.

Olive leaf extract. This all-purpose plant extract has antifungal (anti-Candida), antiviral, and antibacterial properties. It has been successfully used for fibromyalgia, chronic fatigue, sinus infection, parasites, colds, and flu. It is an excellent substitute for antibiotic therapy, as it appears that harmful microorganisms cannot readily develop a resistance to olive leaf extract. (For more information, look for the excellent little book *Olive Leaf Extract,* from the National Life Extension Research Institute, at your health food store).

BR+®. A new herbal complex, BR+®, is a natural solution to microbial and viral ailments, inflammation, immune dysfunction, and free radical damage. The formula combines bloodroot, lesser galangal, olive leaf, aloe vera, and stevia, and the mineral zinc (in the form of zinc picolinate). Only the whole raw roots or leaves are used in this product; no extraction, freezing, or heating is involved. This preserves the potency, bioavailability, inter-herbal synergy, and full range of the plants' multiple bioactive chemistries.

Individually, these ingredients have distinguished histories of safety and efficacy. Bloodroot was listed as a definitive cancer remedy in the

United States Pharmacopoeia from 1820 to 1926. In 1997, German researchers discovered that bloodroot added to animal feed was safer and more effective than antibiotic drugs. Lesser galangal has been a primary herb in Ayurvedic medicine for over 2,000 years. Mediterranean cultures have recognized dozens of healing properties in olive leaf and aloe vera for more than 5,000 years. Prior to stevia's 1903 "discovery" in the Paraguayan jungle, the Guarani Indians had used it as a sweetener and medicine for more than 800 years. As for zinc, it enhances bloodroot's function and has significant therapeutic properties of its own.

Over the last two and a half years, more than 1,000 people have used BR+® successfully for a wide variety of ailments. These results and the scientific literature suggest BR+® can be an effective broad-spectrum preventive, especially for infectious disorders and immune dysfunctions. (For research articles, see the manufacturer's Web site, www.QiVita.net.)

Garlic. Garlic is a natural antimicrobial agent. Excellent for all infections, especially of the lungs and sinuses, garlic has also been used for high blood pressure, parasites, gas, cramps, cancer, contagious diseases, and cholesterol problems. It can be taken in syrup form for all intestinal infections, fevers, flu, stomach problems, ringworm, Candida, and fungal problems. Raw or cooked garlic may be taken with meals. Odorless garlic products are also available. *(Christopher J. The School of Natural Healing. Bi-World Publishers, Provo, UT, 1976.)*

Flaxseed. Flaxseed is exceptional because it contains two of the most significant EFAs: the omega-3 alpha-linolenic acid and the omega-6 linoleic acid. *(Johnston IM, Johnston JR. Flaxseed Oil and the Power of Omega-3. Keats Publishing, New Canaan, CT, 1990.)* A natural laxative, it is also useful for cardiovascular disease as well as inflammation in the digestive tract and joints. Flaxseed oil at a daily dose of 1 tablespoon has been shown to lower blood pressure and cholesterol. You can add crushed flaxseeds to salads, smoothies, and other foods.

S-adenosyl-methionine (SAMe). SAMe is a form of the amino acid methionine, which aids in the brain's production of neurotransmitters and phospholipids (described below). Normally the body produces enough methionine on its own, but this process has been found to be inefficient in depressed individuals. Supplemental SAMe given to depressed people increases their levels of serotonin and dopamine; it acts as an antidepressant in most individuals.

Start with a low dose of 200 milligrams twice daily and increase to 400 milligrams three times daily. *(Rogers SA. Depression: Cured at Last! Sand Key Publishing, Sarasota, FL, 1997.) Caution:* Do not take SAMe if you have bipolar disorder, as this has resulted in serious negative outcomes of anxiety and panic.

Phospholipids. Phospholipids are needed by all cells in the body and are absolutely necessary for normal brain function. Unfortunately, for the past decade or more, we have been convinced that a low-fat diet was the answer—all the while, we have been starving our brain cell membranes.

Phospholipids form double-layered membranes around all cells as well as membranes around the little organelles within cells (mitochondria, nucleus, and lysosomes). Phospholipids help control the passage of many substances (both nutrients and toxins) across these membranes. Phospholipids hold EFAs within the membrane to maintain its fluidity and hold proteins within the membrane to maintain its structure and enable the cell's intake of certain nutrients.

Phospholipids also store the cell's supply of EFAs to attract oxygen, which discourages bacteria, fungi, and viruses from entering. In the bloodstream, phospholipids surround water-soluble vitamins, fats, and cholesterol to prevent them from sticking to each other and keep them moving along. (See the Fats chapter.)

A phospholipid of particular interest is phosphatidylcholine, a component of the nutrient lecithin. It increases levels of the neurotransmitter acetylcholine by providing choline to pair with acetyl molecules. Another, phosphatidylserine, has been used to treat depression and Alzheimer's. Low phosphatidylserine levels are associated with impaired mental function and depression. The brain can manufacture both of these phospholipids if it has enough folic acid and vitamin B$_{12}$.

Phospholipids have been used in the treatment of anxiety, depression, and other mental disorders. Phospholipids are found in foods, but they are not always present in our diet, and they may not be digested properly because of a toxic terrain. In cases of deficiency, they can be taken in supplemental form.

Carnitine. Carnitine is a vitamin-like, vasodilating compound with many functions. The heart and skeletal muscles contain high amounts of carnitine. Epididymal tissues also exhibit high concentrations of carnitine, which is believed to be important for sperm maturation and function.

Carnitine is responsible for transporting fatty acids in the cells and stimulating fat breakdown in the mitochondria. Thus, a deficiency of this compound can reduce energy production, and carnitine concentration is a major factor governing the speed of fat metabolism. Carnitine has been shown to improve blood fat profiles and lower triglyceride levels.

Cardiac muscle derives most (60–80 percent) of its energy from fats, which explains its particularly high content of stored carnitine. A deficiency of carnitine in the heart leads to risk of angina and heart disease. Giving supplemental carnitine to heart patients has relieved angina and improved oxygen uptake from the blood. Carnitine is a bottom-line treatment for heart patients and has also been used to treat respiratory problems. The therapeutic dose for heart and respiratory problems is 1–3 grams daily.

Carnitine is an important supplement for athletes as well. A high level of lactic acid causes fatigue and stiffness, and carnitine's ability to help remove lactic acid from the blood and tissues after exercise is quite significant. It is also linked to the metabolism of branched-chain amino acids (BCAAs), another important consideration for sports performance. (See the Amino Acids chapter.)

A variant called L-acetyl carnitine, manufactured naturally in the brain, is a potent antioxidant and mimics the neurotransmitter acetylcholine. It has been used to delay the progression of Alzheimer's disease and treat depression and age-related memory problems.

5-hydroxytryptophan (5-HTP). A large body of evidence from more than thirty-five years of human and animal studies indicates that supplemental 5-HTP is helpful in a broad range of health problems including depression, anxiety, panic attacks, alcoholism, premenstrual syndrome (PMS), eating disorders, and insomnia. 5-HTP's role is to serve as raw material for synthesis of the neurotransmitter serotonin. Serotonin is used by both the brain and the body. It promotes feelings of calmness, well-being, relaxation, confidence, and security, and in the intestinal tract, serotonin helps regulate peristalsis and digestion.

Because serotonin from the body can't cross the blood-brain barrier, the brain's neurons must make it themselves. Serotonin's precursor tryptophan is consumed through the diet, but it is also used for many other activities in the body, plus it has to compete with other amino acids crossing the blood-brain barrier. Only 1 percent of ingested tryptophan ever reaches the brain, where it is converted to 5-HTP, then to serotonin in the presence of B-vitamins (particularly folic acid and B6). Supplemental 5-HTP, however, can cross the blood-brain barrier for serotonin synthesis.

The suggested way to take supplemental 5-HTP is between meals, away from carbohydrates and proteins, and along with B-vitamins.

Chromium. Chromium is vitally important to health, yet it is very deficient in our diet because of the over-processing of food. A chromium-deficient diet may be an underlying contributor to diabetes, hypoglycemia, insulin resistance, hyperinsulinism, and obesity. (See the Insulin chapter.) Supplementing with chromium can decrease your fasting glucose levels and lower your insulin levels.

Chromium is so important because it's a co-factor for insulin production. It's like a doorkeeper that controls the passage of glucose and other nutrients through the membranes of your 70 trillion cells. If your diet lacks chromium, blood sugar cannot enter your cells for energy production, so it is converted to fat and stored in fat cells.

Chromium controls cells' absorption of amino acids as well. Without it, muscles are not built properly no matter how hard you exercise. (Most people who exercise lose more chromium than people who don't exercise.) Chromium must also be present for cholesterol to enter the cells. If cholesterol stays in the bloodstream instead, it can build up in the vessels, get oxidized, and damage the vessel walls. Studies have shown that restoring chromium in the diet can remove cholesterol deposits.

Although no Recommended Dietary Allowance (RDA) has yet been established for chromium, a daily dose of 200 micrograms appears to be optimal. Chromium picolinate is a well-researched supplement form.

Antioxidants to the Rescue

A few of the most important antioxidants are described below. (Please re-read the chapters on Free Radicals, Phytochemicals, and Fats to get a good understanding of the role that antioxidants play in our diet and health. See also the Juice Plus+® chapter.)

Vitamin E and tocotrienols. Vitamin E is actually a family of eight compounds: alpha, beta, gamma, and delta tocopherols, and alpha, beta, gamma, and delta tocotrienols. Tocotrienols and tocopherols are similar in chemical structure, but tocotrienols are more mobile while tocopherols tend to cluster. Tocopherols (found in corn, soybean, and olive oils) have been used as the standard form of vitamin E; however, new research indicates that tocotrienols (found in palm, rice bran, and barley oils) may be the most important part of the vitamin E spectrum.

One study found that women who took standard vitamin E did not have reduced breast cancer rates, but that women who consumed foods rich in other forms of vitamin E did reduce their risk by 90 percent. Studies have also shown that tocotrienols inhibit the growth of cancer cells. Tocotrienols are powerful against lipid peroxidation, with forty to sixty times the antioxidant effect of alpha tocopherol. Tocotrienols are used for conditions such as atherosclerosis, high cholesterol, and stroke.

As always, try first to eat foods high in vitamin E and tocotrienols before resorting to supplements, as research shows that they're most effective when consumed in whole foods. Sunflower seeds, olives, and almonds are good sources, as are papaya, Swiss chard, spinach, and mustard, turnip, and collard greens. If you choose to supplement, take tocotrienols with meals and in combination with vitamin E.

Co-enzyme Q10 (CoQ10). CoQ10 is a potent antioxidant. Every cell in the body needs CoQ10 to produce energy. It also boosts the immune system's disease-fighting capabilities. A number of studies have shown CoQ10's vital role in the prevention and treatment of many major diseases.

CoQ10 has been called the ignition of the cell, as it has an important function in the cellular manufacture of adenosine triphosphate (ATP), a form of energy that stimulates the cell to perform the metabolic processes supporting its life. With a CoQ10 deficiency, the cellular engine misfires and you experience fatigue. A severe deficiency causes the engine of the cell to fail: no spark, no ignition, no energy, no life.

Dr. Karl Folkers, the father of CoQ10 research, discovered that when levels of this co-enzyme drop below 25 percent of normal, death can occur at the cellular level. He believes that CoQ10 is essential for human life and has theorized that a number of diseases surface when CoQ10 levels drop below 75 percent. *(Folkers K, et al. The activities of coenzyme Q10 and vitamin B6 for immune responses. Biochem Biophys Res Commun 1993 193:88-92.)*

Like vitamin E, CoQ10 protects cell membranes against lipid peroxidation by getting into the phospholipid layer and neutralizing free radicals. Other scientifically reported benefits of CoQ10 are strengthening capillaries, normalizing blood pressure, elevating energy, extending cell life, and being a tonic for the heart. *(Stocker R. Possible health benefits of coenzyme Q10. Linus Pauling Inst Sci Med Newsletter Fall/Winter 2002.)*

Periodontal disease (gum inflammation and degeneration) is a leading cause of tooth loss. In 1970, dentists Raymond F. and Edward G. Wilkinson discovered that adding CoQ10 to the diets of patients with periodontal disease produced measurable improvement in the condition of their gums. *(Wilkinson E, et al. Bioenergetics in clinical medicine VIII. Adjunctive treatment of periodontal disease with co-enzyme Q10. Res Commun Chem Pathol Pharmacol 1976 4:711-719.)* In 1971, Dr. Folkers reported that CoQ10 deficiency causes periodontal disease; other studies confirmed this deficiency in diseased gums. *(Wilkinson E, et al. Bioenergetics in clinical medicine VIII. Adjunctive treatment of periodontal disease with co-enzyme Q10. Res Commun Chem Pathol Pharmacol 1976 4:711-719.)*

CoQ10 can be found in foods such as spinach, broccoli, potatoes, rice, wheat, corn, almonds, and chestnuts. Sometimes, however, it may be necessary to take supplemental CoQ10. Because it is fat-soluble, it is best taken with meals. For heart disease, the usual dose is 300 milligrams daily, whereas a maintenance dose is 90–100 milligrams daily.

Alpha lipoic acid. This antioxidant workhorse is both fat- and water-soluble. Alpha lipoic acid protects cell membranes and helps the body get rid of heavy metals. It has been used by German physicians to treat the tingling of the hands and feet that is a side effect of diabetic neuropathy. Alpha lipoic acid has been shown to stimulate glutathione production in the eye, protecting the lens from cataract formation. It also recycles or regenerates vitamins C and E, CoQ10, and glutathione.

Consider alpha lipoic acid if you are adding antioxidants to your regime, particularly if you are an athlete, as working out produces large amounts of free radicals. For mercury toxicity, take alpha lipoic acid in the range of 300–600 milligrams daily. Take this supplement with meals.

Vitamin C. This vitamin is one of the first lines of antioxidant defense in the watery environment inside and outside of cells. Vitamin C is a preventive against heart disease, stroke, and cancer. It lowers total cholesterol, raises HDL cholesterol, prevents oxidation of LDL cholesterol, and inhibits blood platelet clumping. Vitamin C strengthens and rebuilds collagen tissue and an intercellular material called ground substance; it is good for recovery from all sports injuries as well as for use before and after surgery. It works with the rest of the antioxidants and is also responsible for regenerating vitamin E.

As mentioned for vitamin E, research shows that vitamin C is most effective when consumed within the nutritional complex of whole foods. Some good sources are papaya, red bell peppers, broccoli, Brussels sprouts, strawberries, oranges, kale, and mustard greens.

If you still need additional vitamin C, many supplements are available. Ascorbic acid is the most common type on the market, but you should not take this form if your pH readings are acidic. Instead, take calcium ascorbate or another buffered form or vitamin C esters, which are usually chelated with minerals or substances that have a neutral pH.

A New Kind of Supplement: Whole-Food Concentrates

Over the years, it's been found that not everybody can metabolize megadoses of vitamins and minerals. In fact, megadoses can have the negative effect of stressing the body's systems, especially in chronically ill individuals, because the kidneys and liver must work extra hard to metabolize and eliminate the excess. It is now understood that the value of a supplement is not how much of a nutrient is in the capsule—it's whether you absorb it or not. In most situations, *less is better*. Why bombard your body with excess nutrients if they are not readily absorbed?

Although hundreds of beneficial phytochemicals have been identified, we can be sure that many of the phytochemicals still unknown are very important as well. This underscores the fact that you need plenty of whole foods in your diet. A whole food does not contain a huge amount of any one nutrient—rather, it contains small amounts of numerous nutrients that work together in synergistic balance. By eating whole foods, you bring this synergy into your body. No man-made multinutrient formula can contain all of the vital compounds you need to consume, because metabolically necessary nutrients are yet to be discovered and because it is impossible to re-create nature's synergy in a laboratory.

This is why so many bioavailable whole-food concentrates, created by companies such as NSA, Inc., are appearing on the health food scene today. (See the Juice Plus+® chapter.)

JUICE PLUS+®: THE MOST RESEARCHED NUTRACEUTICAL IN THE WORLD TODAY

Before I tell you about the research behind Juice Plus+®, I'd like to tell you the personal story that led to the development of this whole-food product. When we're experiencing a trauma or other significant event, we don't always fully understand it until it has passed, and then we realize that it has changed our lives for the better. Living a life is a lesson itself and is always teaching us something; we just have to learn how to interpret the direction it is taking us. Even a chronic illness is pointing us in a specific direction, as I learned when my father got sick.

It was 1980 and I was on a lecture tour, teaching herbal seminars in Denver, Colorado. During a break, I received a phone call from my father. He told me his spleen had swollen to the size of a football. It was so large he was using one of his Marine Corp belts to hold it up and it was so painful that he could hardly move. My mother made an appointment for him at a nearby hospital, where the doctors could not believe how large his spleen had grown—and it was still growing.

At the end of the day, my dad called me again and said he was diagnosed with lymphoma, cancer of the lymphatic system. I was so stunned I couldn't even reply. I just held the phone, praying that I didn't really hear what he had said. My throat closed up, so tight I could hardly breathe. He felt my shock and distress and told me everything was going to be okay. Being a naturopath and teaching people for years how to live by the laws of nature, I had to ask myself, why did this have to happen? (Don't we all wonder why, when something so traumatic happens to us?)

I told my dad I'd be home in four days as soon as my tour was over. By the time I got there, his doctors had already removed his spleen and started chemotherapy. I was floored, totally irate. No questions had been asked—they just did the surgery and started pumping him full of drugs.

After three weeks, my father had lost 40 pounds and nothing was working. The chemotherapy had failed and there was nothing more they could do. His doctor called our family together and told us my dad had no more than three weeks to live. After breaking the news to my dad, I asked if he'd like to try natural therapy at my clinic in Tucson, where I would take care of him. He said, "I would have come to you before this, but I didn't want you to be responsible if anything bad would have happened to me." I picked him up and carried him out of the hospital without even checking him out.

By the time we got to Tucson, he weighed 136 pounds, and his cancer was traveling so fast through his body that he couldn't eat or drink. How do you nourish somebody who can't eat or drink? I started massaging him every day with olive oil so his body would absorb the fat through his skin. He could only sip water, so I devised a plan to get more nutrients in through another route. I built a slant board for him to lie on, made fresh green juice with kale, parsley, and some additional liquid chlorophyll, and used an enema bag to feed him through the bowel with this juice daily.

As he got stronger, he was able to drink vegetable juices by mouth. Fruit juices, however, made him feel ill because of their sugar. You don't want to feed cancer cells sugar, because they thrive on it; plus, it acidifies the body, putting an even greater strain on a sick person's system.

I wanted to find a way to get more concentrated nutrition into his body to increase his strength and boost his healing, and it occurred to me that if I could juice the vegetables and dry the juice, the powder would be more concentrated than the juice itself. I set up some small dryers in my office and found that it would take hours to dry the juice, but it worked. I'd give him tablespoons of vegetable juice powder stirred into small amounts of water daily. To my amazement—keep in mind, at that time we knew nothing about phytochemicals—in two months he put on 30 pounds. There was no meat or carbohydrates other than tablespoons of dried vegetable juice in his diet. I wondered, how could someone put on so much weight without eating?

He then got to the point where he could also drink fruit juice powder without feeling ill, so he'd have fruit juice powder in the morning and vegetable juice powder the rest of the day. I gave him very little fruit juice powder, though, as I noticed that if I gave him too much, his urine's pH would turn acidic. I also added proteolytic enzymes and some herbs to the regime. I was constantly changing the dosages of his supplements according to his pH, using the monitoring system in this book.

The results were astonishing. Within three months of my taking over his treatment, my father got out of bed and remodeled my kitchen. He had been a carpenter his whole life and loved working with wood. Continuing on a nutritional program of eating large amounts of vegetables, dried juice powders, and soaked and sprouted seeds and nuts, he went back to work within six months and worked as a carpenter for another six years. It's my opinion that he'd still be alive today if his doctors had not removed his spleen and given him such high doses of drugs during his hospitalization.

From my father's recovery, I realized the hidden healing power of whole foods, so I began studying all fruits and vegetables known to man, and discovered that some were much more nutrient-dense than others. The ones most concentrated in nutrients were the ones most people didn't eat at all, or always cooked before eating: parsley, beets, cabbage, and broccoli, to name a few. Experimenting with several fruits and vegetables over several months, I designed one concentrated powder formula with fruits and another with vegetables. These two formulas contained the most nutrient-dense fruits and vegetables on the planet.

By this time my clinic looked more like a drying facility for fruit and vegetable juice powders, and everyone who came to me, regardless of the problem, was given a bag of each powder. The healings that I observed were no less than miraculous. I knew I was on to something big when my patients were getting well so fast. I quickly contacted a patent attorney but it took five years to get the patent on my idea, which I received on my birthday. That was significant to me because I believe that everything that happens to us is God-sent, a gift to receive and learn from.

The formulas that I used for those years in my clinical practice are now called Juice Plus+®. I designed and patented this product, and NSA, Inc. in Memphis, TN manufactured, distributed, and promoted it. Today, these God-given products are benefiting thousands of people in over thirty countries.

Just before my father died, he was so concerned about my professional reputation that he said, "If I die, will people still believe in you? Will they still buy your books?" I said, "Dad, what we accomplished together, this idea of concentrated fruits and vegetables, someday will be known all over the world." And that's exactly what happened. My father's recovery gave birth to the most wonderful product line of fruit and vegetable concentrates, Juice Plus+®.

My father taught me pride and honor. He would tell me that a man's word is all he has. In over fifty years of being a carpenter, he never once had a written contract with anyone—only an agreement of a smile, honor, and love. He will always own a piece of my heart. I know he is always with me; he's my strength and motivation.

The Research Behind Juice Plus+®

I'd like to give special thanks and appreciation to NSA's corporate family and distributors for believing in me and the concept of Juice Plus+®, especially President Jay Martin and Vice President John Blair, who are totally responsible for the marketing, research, and distribution of these products. Thanks also go to Jeff Roberti, who introduced me to NSA and was the first person to acknowledge the validity of this concept.

Numerous clinical studies published in peer-reviewed scientific journals have demonstrated the following benefits of Juice Plus+®:

Juice Plus+® delivers key phytonutrients that are easily absorbed by the body. Several studies have shown the bioavailability of select nutrients found in Juice Plus+® in a variety of populations. At Tokyo Women's Medical University, Juice Plus+® was shown to increase the bioavailability of various nutrients in a Japanese population. *(Kawashima A, et al. Four week supplementation with mixed fruit and vegetable juice concentrates increased protective serum antioxidants and folate and decreased plasma homocysteine in Japanese subjects. Asia Pacific J Clin Nutr 2007 16:411-421.)* The bioavailability of Juice Plus+® was also demonstrated in studies in Europe (Medical University Vienna and King's College London) and Australia (University of Sydney). *(Kiefer L, et al. Supplementation with mixed fruit and vegetable juice concentrates increased serum antioxidants and folate in healthy adults. J Am Coll Nutr 2004 23:205-211; Leeds AR, et al. Availability of micronutrients from dried, encapsulated fruit and vegetable preparations: a study in healthy volunteers. J Hum Nutr Dietetics 2000 13:21-27; Samman S, et al. A mixed fruit and vegetable concentrate increases plasma antioxidant vitamins and folate and lowers plasma homocysteine in men. J Nutr 2003 133:2188-2193.)*

In the United States, the bioavailability of Juice Plus+® has been shown in young adults (University of Florida), middle-aged people (Vanderbilt University School of Medicine) and the elderly (University of Texas Health Science Center). *(Nantz MP, et al. Immunity and antioxidant capacity in humans is enhanced by consumption of a dried, encapsulated fruit and vegetable juice concentrate. J Nutr 2006 136:2606-2610; Houston MC, et al. Juice powder concentrate and systemic blood pressure, progression of coronary artery calcium and antioxidant status in hypertensive subjects: a pilot study. Evidence-Based Compl Alt Med 2007 doi:10.1093/ecam/nel108; Wise JA, et al. Changes in plasma carotenoids, alpha-tocopherol, and lipid peroxide levels in response to supplementation with concentrated fruit and vegetable extracts: a pilot study. Curr Ther Res 1996 57:445-461.)*

Juice Plus+® reduces oxidative stress. Several investigations have reported that Juice Plus+® reduced various markers (signs) of oxidative stress. A study at the University of North Carolina-Greensboro showed that Juice Plus+® Orchard, Garden, and Vineyard Blends together were effective in reducing a marker of oxidative stress associated with aerobic exercise. *(Bloomer RJ, et al. Oxidative stress response to aerobic exercise: comparison of antioxidant supplements. Med Sci Sports Ex 2006 38:1098-1105.)* Improvements in other markers of oxidative stress have been noted in studies of sedentary people in the United States (University of Texas Health Science Center) and England (King's College London). *(Wise JA, et al. Changes in plasma carotenoids, alpha-tocopherol, and lipid peroxide levels in response to supplementation with concentrated fruit and vegetable extracts: a pilot study. Curr Ther Res 1996 57:445-461; Leeds AR, et al. Availability of micronutrients from dried, encapsulated fruit and vegetable preparations: a study in healthy volunteers. J Human Nutr Dietetics 2000 13:21-27.)*

Juice Plus+® helps support a healthy immune system. A healthy immune system protects the body, and good nutrition is critical for a healthy immune system. Clinical studies showed that Juice Plus+® improved several measures of immune function in young adult students at the University of Florida and in elderly people at the University of Arizona. *(Nantz MP, et al. Immunity and antioxidant capacity in humans is enhanced by consumption of a dried, encapsulated fruit and vegetable juice concentrate. J Nutr 2006 136:2606-2610; Inserra PF, et al. Immune function in elderly smokers and nonsmokers improves during supplementation with fruit and vegetable extracts. Integr Med 1999 2:3-10.)*

Juice Plus+® helps protect DNA. DNA becomes damaged and fragile when exposed to oxidative stress; a high-quality diet rich in fruits and vegetables (and their antioxidants) helps protect DNA from oxidative damage that can weaken its structural integrity. Studies showed a reduction in DNA damage after taking Juice Plus+® in both young adults (University of Florida) and in an elderly population (Brigham Young University). *(Nantz MP, et al. Immunity and antioxidant capacity in humans is enhanced by consumption of a dried, encapsulated fruit and vegetable juice concentrate. J Nutr 2006 136:2606-2610; Smith MJ, et al. Supplementation with fruit and vegetable extracts may decrease DNA damage in the peripheral lymphocytes of an elderly population. Nutr Res 1999 19:1507-1518.)*

Juice Plus+® positively affects several key indicators of cardiovascular wellness. Several investigations have found that Juice Plus+® reduces homocysteine levels. A clinical study at the University of Sydney showed a reduction of homocysteine levels in participants whose levels were already within an acceptable range. *(Samman S, et al. A mixed fruit and vegetable concentrate increases plasma antioxidant vitamins and folate and lowers plasma homocysteine in men. J Nutr 2003 133:2188-2193.)* Researchers in Foggia, Italy found that Juice Plus+® reduced homocysteine levels in participants whose levels had been elevated. *(Panunzio MF, et al. Supplementation with fruit and vegetable concentrate decreases plasma homocysteine in a dietary controlled trial. Nutr Res 2003 23:1221-1228.)* Researchers at the University of Maryland found that participants who consumed Juice Plus+® were better able to maintain elasticity of their arteries, even after a high-fat meal. *(Plotnick GD, et al. Effect of supplemental phytonutrients on impairment of the flow-mediated brachial artery vasoactivity after a single high-fat meal. J Am Coll Cardiol 2003 41:1744-1749.)* Investigators at Vanderbilt University School of Medicine monitored several measures of vascular health in a low-risk population who took Juice Plus+® for two years, and noted modest improvements with no adverse side effects. *(Houston MC, et al. Juice powder concentrate and systemic blood pressure, progression of coronary artery calcium and antioxidant status in hypertensive subjects: a pilot study. Evidence-Based Compl Alt Med 2007 doi:10.1093/ecam/nel108.)*

Examples of current and past Juice Plus+® research affiliations:
Brigham Young University
Georgetown University
King's College, London, England
Medical University of Graz, Austria
Medical University of Vienna, Austria
Tokyo Women's Medical University, Japan
University of Arizona
University of Birmingham, England
University of California, Los Angeles
University of Florida
University of Maryland School of Medicine
University of Milan, Italy
University of Mississippi Medical Center
University of North Carolina-Greensboro
University of South Carolina
University of Sydney, Australia
University of Texas Health Science Center
University of Texas/MD Anderson
University of Würzburg, Germany
Vanderbilt University School of Medicine
Wake Forest University (with the NCI-National Institutes of Health)
Yale University-Griffin Hospital Prevention Research Center

(For more information on the clinical research conducted on Juice Plus+®, please visit www.JuicePlus.com.)

A FINAL WORD FROM DR. SANTILLO

Is there really Alternative Medicine? There is no Alternative Medicine. The body-power within does the healing. Whether you favor drugs or herbs—both are necessary. Both work by helping and assisting the body to heal itself. When the body expresses symptoms, it's speaking to you, saying there is some kind of imbalance. Use whatever is absolutely necessary to bring it back into balance. But always support it with a good diet and whole-food supplement.

It's the promiscuous use of both drugs and supplements that causes other symptomologies, not one or the other. Do not separate the healing arts. Let's all work together. Nothing on this planet is separate. Our job as healers is to assist humanity with the truth, not tear it apart with opinions. Knowledge is the greatest weapon on earth.

I had my internship with a man who was a medical doctor and a naturopath. He used drugs when necessary and herbs when need be. He blurred the line between "us" and "them." Because there is no line, no us and them—just knowledge, understanding, progress, and the hope that someday we'll all work together. There are too many people sick in this world to say that one type of doctor, philosophy, or theory has all the answers. Tap into the wisdom of the body; the spirit within has all the answers. Given that we have trillions of cells in our bodies and each cell performs hundreds of functions a second, where do you think the wisdom lies: in an herb or drug? Support the wisdom within and love your body. It's a precious gift, and it's not permanent.

There is nothing alternative about healing. The laws of the body are the same now as they've ever been. Good nutrition, exercise, controlled emotions, look for the good and go about doing good, be at peace—these are the laws we must obey. It's always been this way. If you're not antagonistic about anything, then there is no alternative. How can anything be alternative to natural law? There is no exception or division in natural law. The seasons are the seasons, so we live, we die—the laws of life dictate. You all have a religion or philosophy you believe in; you can't change it, you can only live it the best you can. Do you think there's an alternative to that?

Take it easy, and enjoy your life, your family, and your friends. The jewels of life are within you and so is healing. I wish you wellness, happiness, and a wonderful future. Thank you for spending your precious time reading this book. God bless.

ADDITIONAL REFERENCES

Balch JF, Balch PA. *Prescription for Nutritional Healing*. Avery Publishing Group, Garden City Park, NY, 1997.

Bernard S, et al. Autism: a novel form of mercury poisoning. *Med Hypotheses* 2001 564:462-471.

Borek C. *Maximize Your Health-Span with Antioxidants*. Keats Publishing, New Canaan, CT, 1995.

Buist R. *Food Chemical Sensitivity*. Avery Publishing Group, Garden City Park, NY, 1988.

Chaitow L. *Thorson's Guide to Amino Acids*. Harper Collins Publishing, London, UK, 1991.

Colagiuri S. *The New Glucose Revolution*. Marlowe and Company, New York, NY, 2003.

Colgan M. *Optimum Sports Nutrition*. Advanced Research Press, New York, NY, 1993.

Diet, nutrition and the prevention of chronic diseases. A report of the WHO study on diet, nutrition and prevention of non-communicable diseases. *Nutr Rev* 1991 49:291-301.

DiPasquale M. *Amino Acids and Proteins for the Athlete*. CRC Press, Boca Raton, FL, 1997.

Eades MR, Eades MD. *The Protein Power Life Plan*. Warner Books, New York, NY, 2000.

Erdmann R. *The Amino Revolution*. Simon and Schuster, New York, NY, 1987.

Fallon S, Enig MG. *Nourishing Traditions*. New Trends Publishing, Washington DC, 1999.

Firshein R. *The Nutraceutical Revolution*. Riverhead Books, New York, NY, 1998.

Gittleman AL. *Beyond Pritikin*. Bantam Books, New York, NY, 1996.

Guyton AC. *Function of the Human Body*. W.B Saunders Company, Philadelphia, PA, 1974.

Herman C, et al. Soybean phytoestrogen intake and cancer risk. *J Nutr* 1995 125:757S-770S.

Kennedy AR. The evidence for soybean products as cancer preventive agents. *J Nutr* 1995 125:733S-743S.

Kihara T, et al. Repeated sauna treatment improves vascular endothelial and cardiac function in patients with chronic heart failure. *J Am Coll Cardiol* 2002 39:754-759.

Klatz R, Goldman R. *Stopping the Clock.*. Bantam Books, New York, NY, 1996.

Kristal HJ. *The Nutrition Solution.* North Atlantic Books, Berkeley, CA, 2002.

Lampe JW, et al. Urinary lignan and isoflavonoid excretion in premenopausal women consuming flaxseed powder. *Am J Clin Nutr* 1994 60:122-128.

Lark SM, Richards JA. *The Chemistry of Success.* Bay Books, San Francisco, CA, 2000.

Meletis CD. *Interactions Between Drugs and Natural Medicines.* Eclectic Medical Publications, Sandy, OR, 1999.

Mercola J, Levy AR. *The No-Grain Diet.* Dutton, New York, NY, 2003.

Moore M. *Medicinal Plants of the Mountain West.* Museum of New Mexico Press, Santa Fe, NM, 1979.

Oelke J. *Natural Choices for Fibromyalgia.* Natural Choices, St. Joseph, MI, 2002.

Papas AM. *Antioxidant Status, Diet, Nutrition, and Health.* CRC Press, Boca Raton, FL, 1999.

Rogers SA. *Pain Free in 6 Weeks.* Sand Key Company, Sarasota, FL, 2001.

Ross J. *The Diet Cure.* Viking, New York, NY, 1999.

Santillo H. *Food Enzymes: The Missing Link to Radiant Health.* Hohm Press, Prescott, AZ, 1993.

Santillo H. *Intuitive Eating.* Hohm Press, Prescott, AZ, 1993.

Santillo H. *Natural Healing with Herbs.* Hohm Press, Prescott, AZ, 1993.

Schimmel HW. *Functional Medicine.* Haug Verlag, Heidelberg, Germany, 1997.

Silver N. *The Handbook of Rife Frequency Healing.* Center for Frequency Education, Stone Ridge, NY, 2001.

Stoll AL. *The Omega-3 Connection.* Simon and Schuster, New York, NY, 2001.

Thompson LU. Potential health benefits of whole grains and their components. *Contemp Nutr* 1992 17:1-2.

Wolcott WL, Fahey T. *The Metabolic Typing Diet.* Doubleday, New York, NY, 2000.

Wolf M, Ransberger K. *Enzyme Therapy.* Regent House, Los Angeles, CA, 1977.

Young RO, Young SR. *The pH Miracle.* Warner Books, New York, NY, 2002.

INDEX

insulin resistance, 101–102
insult, 55–56
intellectual sluggishness, 184
intelligent rejectivity, 59
intelligent selectivity, 59
interconnectedness of body tissues, 19
internal/interior environment, 33, 35, 54, 57, 58, 63, 112, 138–139
intoxication, 61–62
iodine, 73, 99, 106, 110–111, 137, 147, 178
ionic minerals, 103
IQ tests, 191
iron, 50, 161
irritability, 62, 164
irritable bowel syndrome, 28, 136, 188, 231, 279
islets of Langerhans, 202
isoleucine, 185, 210
isopathic therapy, 53
Itano, Pawling, 37

J

Jacob, S., 286
Jenson, Karen, 282
Johnson, B.E., 156
joint degeneration, 157
Joint Health, 287
Juice Plus+®, 12, 83–84, 95–96, 102, 141, 153, 155, 210, 141, 155, 210, 264–265, 278, 285, 304–311
juices, 102, 112, 177
junk foods, 266
junk-food diet, 203

K

kale, 148
Kasai, K., 192
Kawashima, A., 308
kelp, 102
Kidney Liquid, 95
kidneys
    acidic waste and, 50, 72–73, 75, 86, 95
    cadmium and, 163
    circulation and, 257
    damage by NSAIDs, 136
    dandelion root/leaf and, 291

dental mercury and, 164
detoxification, 104
excess protein and, 262
glucose and, 198
glutamine and, 189
heavy metal toxicity and, 161, 166
high carbohydrate diet and, 204
hormone imbalance and, 27–28
linoleic acid (LA) and, 213
potassium and, 117
respiration and, 227
sodium and, 101, 128
whole-food concentrates and, 303
Kiefer, L., 308
Klatz, Ronald, 193–194
Kulvinskas, Viktoras, 245

L

Lachesis, 125
lack of ambition, 79
lactic acid waste, 49, 50, 51, 79
Lactobacillus acidophilus, 112, 284
law of rejectivity, 54
law of selectivity, 54
Lawrence, R., 286
L-carnitine, 125
LDLs (low-density lipoproteins), 152–153, 199
L-dopa, 184, 293–294
lead, 163–164
lead lines, 164
Leaf, Alexander, 228–229
leafy green vegetables, 271
leaky bowel syndrome, 65, 237
leaky gut syndrome, 136–139
learning difficulties, 158
Lee, Lita, 286
Leeds, A.R., 308, 309
lesser galangal, 294–295
leucine, 185, 210
leukemia, 49, 161, 164
levodopa, 294
Lexotan, 188
libido, low/loss of, 160, 187
Librium, 188